F. M. J. Debruyne R. M. Bukowski
J. E. Pontes P. H. M. de Mulder (Eds.)

Immunotherapy of Renal Cell Carcinoma

Clinical and Experimental Developments

With the Assistance of R. J. A. van Moorselaar

With Contributions by
R. Ackermann J. Alexander Y. Aso T.T. Back
B. Barna A. J. M. C. Beniers J. P. Bergerat C. Bollack
J. Boyett G. T. Budd R. M. Bukowski F. Corrado G. Corrado
F. M. J. Debruyne C. De Vinci M. J. Droller P. Dufour I. J. Fidler
J. Finke J. Ford S. D. Fosså M. P. H. Franssen H. Futami
V. Gibson R. Heicappell R. Herbrecht R. L. Hornung
D. Jacqmin J. Jurascheck Y. Kakehi J. J. Killion
E. A. Klein W. M. Linehan K. Marumo C. S. McCune
S. Medendorp R. J. A. van Moorselaar P. H. M. de Mulder
S. Murthy F. Oberling G. Pizza J. E. Pontes G. Prevost
C. J. A. Punt P. Rayman P. Salze T. J. Sayers J. A. Schalken
J. Sergi H. Tazaki R. Tubbs T. Umeda R. L. Vessella
R. H. Wiltrout M. P. Wirth O. Yoshida H. A. Young

Springer-Verlag
Berlin Heidelberg New York
London Paris Tokyo
Hong Kong Barcelona

Frans M. J. Debruyne, MD, Ph. D.
Director and Chairman, Department of Urology
University Hospital Nijmegen
P. O. Box 9101, 6500 HB Nijmegen, The Netherlands

Ronald M. Bukowski, MD
Director, Clinical Research, Cleveland Clinic Cancer Center
Cleveland Clinic Foundation
9500 Euclid Avenue, Cleveland, Ohio 44106, USA

J. Edson Pontes, MD, Ph. D.
Professor and Chairman, Department of Urology
Wayne State University
4160 John R., Suite 1017, Detroit, Michigan 48201, USA

Pieter H. M. de Mulder, MD, Ph. D.
Department of Medical Oncology
University Hospital Nijmegen
P. O. Box 9101, 6500 HB Nijmegen, The Netherlands

With 20 Figures

ISBN-13:978-3-540-52835-7 e-ISBN-13:978-3-642-75853-9
DOI: 10.1007/978-3-642-75853-9

10/3130-543210 – Printed on acid-free paper

Preface

New interesting clinical and scientific developments in the immunotherapeutic management of renal cell carcinoma have been achieved in the past years. Since BRM's such as Interferon became available in a larger scale in the early eighties, many clinical and fundamental researchers have been stimulated to investigate not only their efficacy in direct patient care but also to elucidate their mechanism of action and how to improve their effects. This research is still in its earliest stages and it has to be expected that further developments and improved insight in this complicated field will be achieved in the coming years.

Scientists are used to communicate their research, and the results and hypotheses originating from it, in scientific journals or at large or small scale scientific meetings, congresses, symposia or workshops. Two most interesting meetings on the experimental and clinical progress in the immunological management of renal cell carcinoma have been organized recently in Europe (Nijmegen, the Netherlands) and the USA (Cleveland, Ohio). The organizers of these meetings have been stimulated by the participating experts to publish the interesting data discussed. The response to our requests to the lecturers and moderators to send in a manuscript of the work they presented and discussed has resulted in this monograph on immunotherapy of renal cell carcinoma. It will provide the interested reader with up to date information on the developments and innovations in this field. General overviews and detailed experimental research are discussed in various chapters, providing general information, but also indicating the directions for future developments.

We sincerely want to thank all contributors for their discipline in submitting the manuscripts and the high quality of their work.

We also want to thank Dr. R. J. A. van Moorselaar for his critical, but excellent help in preparing the manuscripts for publication. The expertise of Springer has guaranteed the highest technical quality. We wish all readers interesting and stimulating moments while reading and/or consulting this monograph.

F. D.
R. B.
E. P.
P. M.

Contents

Clinical Experience with Biological Response Modifiers in Renal Cell Carcinoma

List of Contributors

Addresses are given at the beginning of the respective contribution.

Introduction

W.M. Linehan[1]

Renal cell carcinoma, the most common neoplasm in the kidney, occurs in 23 000 people annually in the United States and is responsible for over 10 000 deaths annually. The 2-year survival rate for patients with advanced renal cell carcinoma is only 10%–15%; there are currently no effective standard therapies available for patients with this disease. Recently there have been a number of exciting developments in the understanding of both the molecular and cellular events associated with transformation in renal cell carcinoma as well as in new forms of immunological therapy for patients with advanced forms of this malignancy.

The initial study evaluating chromosomal abnormalities associated with renal cell carcinoma, by Cohen et al. demonstrated a translocation from chromosome 3 to chromosome 8 in affected family members with familial renal cell carcinoma [1]. A subsequent study in another kindred with a familial form of renal cell carcinoma revealed a chromosome 3 to chromosome 11 translocation in tumor tissue from a patient with this disease [5]. These studies led to the use of the molecular technique of restriction fragment polymorphism analysis, which detected loss of hererozygosity on the short arm of chromosome 3 in tumor tissue from patients with the sporadic form of renal cell carcinoma, suggesting the presence of a disease gene or tumor suppressor gene at this location [4, 14]. Subsequent studies detected this same molecular abnormality in renal tumors from patients with a familial form of renal cell carcinoma associated with von Hippel-Lindau disease [12]. These and other studies demonstrated that there is a disease gene on the short arm of chromosome 3 which is thought to be associated with the initiation and/or progression of renal cell carcinoma. The recent study demonstrating that introduction of a normal chromosome 3 back into renal cell carcinoma can inhibit tumor growth in xenografts and significantly alter in vitro characteristics [10] suggests that isolation of the gene on chromosome 3 responsible for human renal cell carcinoma may enable investigators not only to understand the molecular events associated with this disease but also to potentially develop new forms of therapy for this malignancy.

Recent studies of the cellular abnormalities associated with renal cell carcinoma have demonstrated abnormalities both in growth factors and growth factor receptors, as well as the multidrug resistance gene in kidney cancer. Kidney cancer has been shown to be associated with an increased expression of the transforming

[1] Urologic Oncology Section, Surgery Branch, National Institutes of Health, Building 10, Bethesda, MD 20892, USA

F.M.J. Debruyne et al. (Eds.)
Immunotherapy of Renal Cell Carcinoma

growth factor TGF-α and also with its receptor, the EGF receptor [3, 9]. These together with similar studies reported in this monograph raise the possibility that there may be autocrine stimulation of renal cell carcinoma by a tumor-produced growth factor such as TGF-α. Therapeutic strategies involving monoclonal antibodies and other cytotoxic agents targeted at these growth factors and at growth factor receptors are currently being developed. Fojo and others have demonstrated that there is an increased expression of the MDR1 gene in human renal cell carcinoma [2]. The MDR1 gene product, P-glycoprotein, is thought to play a role in the chemoresistance of this tumor. Clinical strategies aimed at reversing expression of this gene in order to develop more effective chemotherapeutic regimens for treatment are currently being evaluated in preclinical as well as clinical trials [13].

A new strategy for treatment of patients with advanced renal cell carcinoma with adoptive immunotherapy has recently been developed in the Surgery Branch of the National Cancer Institute (NCI). Adoptive immunotherapy involves the transfer to the tumor host of active immunologic reagents with antitumor activity. An initial form of this therapy involved interleukin-2 (IL-2) and lymphokine-activated killer cells (LAK). Rosenberg and co-workers demonstrated that both IL-2 alone and IL-2 + LAK have antitumor activity in patients with advanced renal cell carcinoma [6]. In the NCI clinical trials, 35% of patients with advanced renal cell carcinoma displayed a complete or partial response to therapy with IL-2 + LAK [7]. In an attempt to develop a more effective therapeutic strategy for patients with this malignancy, studies utilizing the combination of IL-2 plus other biologic agents such as interferon [8], as well as attempts to identify a more potent cell for adoptive therapy such as the tumor-infiltrating lymphocytes [11], have been initiated. Currently, investigators are evaluating the use of combinations of lymphokines with other biologic agents as well as chemotherapeutic agents in the treatment of patients with kidney cancer.

As this monograph demonstrates, collaborative projects involving urologic and oncologic surgeons, medical oncologists, radiation oncologists and basic scientists studying the basic and clinical aspects of renal cell carcinoma are ongoing at a number of medical centers around the world. Hopefully, new developments in our understanding of the cellular and molecular events associated with transformation in renal cell carcinoma as well as advances in new forms of immunologic therapy will lead to an effective form of therapy for patients with this malignancy.

References

1. Cohen AJ, Li FP, Berg S, Marchetto DJ, Tsai S, Jacobs SC, Brown RS (1979) Hereditary renal-cell carcinoma associated with a chromosomal translocation. N Engl J Med 301:592–595
2. Fojo AJ, Ueda K, Slamon DJ, Poplack DG, Gottesman MM, Pastan I (1987) Expression of a multidrug-resistance gene in human tumors and tissues. Proc Natl Acad Sci USA 84:265–269

3. Gomella LG, Sargent ER, Wade TP, Anglard P, Linehan WM, Kasid A (1989) Expression of transforming growth factor alpha in normal human adult kidney and enhanced expression of transforming growth factors alpha and beta 1 in renal cell carcinoma. Cancer Res 49:6972–6975
4. Linehan M, Miller E, Anglard P, Merino M, Zbart B (1989) Improved detection of allele loss in renal cell carcinomas after removal of leukocytes by immunologic selection. J Natl Cancer Inst 81:287–290
5. Pathak S, Strong LC, Ferrell RE, Trindade A (1982) Familial renal cell carcinoma with a 3;11 chromosome translocation limited to tumor cells. Science 217:939–941
6. Rosenberg SA, Lotze MT, Muul Lm, Chang AE, Avis FP, Leitman S, Linehan WM et al. (1987) A progress report on the treatment of 157 patients with advanced cancer using lymphokine-activated killer cells and interleukin-2 or high-dose interleukin-2 alone. N Engl Med 316:889–897
7. Rosenberg SA, Lotze MT, Yang JC, Aebersold PM, Linehan WM, Seipp CA, White DE (1989) Experience with the use of high-dose interleukin-2 in the treatment of 652 cancer patients. Ann Surg 210:474–484
8. Rosenberg SA, Lotze MT, Yang JC, Linehan WM, Seipp C, Calabro S, Karp SE et al. (1989) Combination therapy with interleukin-2 and alpha-interferon for the treatment of patients with advanced cancer. J Clin Oncol 7:1863–1874
9. Sargent ER, Gomella LG, Belldegrun A, Linehan WM, Kasid A (1989) Epidermal growth factor receptor gene expression in normal human kidney and renal cell carcinoma. J Urol 142:1364–1368
10. Shimizu M, Yokota J, Mori N, Shuin T, Shinoda M, Terada M, Oshimura M (1990) Introduction of normal chromosome 3p modulates the tumorigenicity of a human renal cell carcinoma cell line YCR. Oncogene 5:185–194
11. Topalian SL, Solomon D, Avis FP, Chang AE, Freerksen DL, Linehan WM, Lotze MT et al. (1988) Immunotherapy of patients with advanced cancer using tumor-infiltrating lymphocytes and recombinant interleukin-2: a pilot study. J Clin Oncol 6:839–853
12. Tory K, Brauch H, Linehan M, Barba D, Oldfield E, Filling-Katz M, Seizinger B et al. (1989) Specific genetic change in tumors associated with von Hippel-Lindau disease. J Natl Cancer Inst 81:1097–1101
13. Weiss GH, McAtee N, Mickley L, Robertson CN, Gottesmann MM, Pastan IH, Linehan WM, Fojo T (1990) Clinical trial of amiodarone to suppress function of multidrug resistance gene product during chemotherapy for renal cell carcinoma. J Urol 143 (4):385A:
14. Zbar B, Brauch H, Talmadge C, Linehan M (1987) Loss of alleles of loci on the short arm of chromosome 3 in renal cell carcinoma. Nature 327:721–724

Experimental Data

Considerations in Immunotherapy of Genitourinary Neoplasia

M. J. Droller[1]

Introduction

Cancer immunotherapy encompasses the need to understand the fundamentals of tumor biology, immune response mechanisms, experimental and applied immunotherapy, and the design and assessment of clinical trials. Each of these areas is highly complex. Notwithstanding the major strides that have been made in our knowledge, the role of immunotherapy in the treatment of cancer remains both unclear and controversial.

This discussion is not intended as an exhaustive review of cancer immunotherapy. Rather, I shall present some of the principles within each of the relevant areas that form the basis of our understanding. As such, this overview is intended to provide a background upon which the other discussions related to immunotherapy in this monograph can be placed.

The Immune Response in Cancer

The immune response constitutes a highly specific cellular or humoral reaction to a particular molecule (antigen) that is recognized as foreign by the host. Although the immune response has traditionally been separated into humoral (antibody) and cellular compartments, it actually consists of a complex network of interactions that induce, stimulate, or inhibit the activities of the individual components in each section. The general response involves antigen recognition by particular cells, antigen processing, activation of various types of lymphocytes that respond to presentation of processed antigens, and resultant cellular interactions that then generate activity against the foreign molecule. In tumor immunology, this sequence involves macrophage recognition of putative tumor-associated antigens, their processing and presentation to various types of T lymphocytes, activation and proliferation of specific subpopulations of B and T lymphocytes, antibody production, generation of cytotoxic effector cells [T lymphocytes, natural killer (NK) cells, killer (K) cells, and macrophages], and production of lymphokines and cytokines that either amplify or inhibit the specific immune response.

[1] Department of Urology, The Mount Sinai Medical Center, New York, NY 10029-6574, USA

F.M.J. Debruyne et al. (Eds.)
Immunotherapy of Renal Cell Carcinoma

A tumor cell can only initiate an immune response if it has the capacity for immunogenicity. It must first be recognized by the host as foreign. It must present antigens that can be taken up by macrophages and processed. The processed antigen then needs to be recognized by helper T lymphocytes which will assist in the generation of cytotoxic T lymphocytes and antibodies. Recognition is determined not only by the foreignness of an antigen but also by the compatibility of the major histocompatibility complexes shared between the stimulatory and reactive cells. The efficacy of various cellular interactions is critical for tumor immunogenicity to be expressed.

A variety of molecules are important in the stimulation and regulation of these cellular interactions. When helper T lymphocytes bind to the macrophage-processed tumor antigen, they produce interleukin-2 (IL-2) and gamma interferon (IFNγ). IL-2 induces the generation of other helper T cells and killer T cells. The helper T cells induce B cells to multiply and produce antibodies. The killer T cells are programmed to attack those cells that have expressed the antigens that initiated the response. Macrophages produce IL-1 and tumor necrosis factor (TNF). TNF may act on the vascular supply of the tumor bed. IL-1 stimulates T lymphocytes to produce additional IL-2 which leads to further generation of helper and cytotoxic T lymphocytes. In addition, receptors to IL-2 are induced on NK cells, which respond by proliferation and increased activity. Each of these cells also secretes IL-2, thereby leading to a self-generating or autocrine function. The NK cells together with the helper T lymphocytes also produce IFNγ, which stimulates macrophages, cytotoxic T lymphocytes, and NK cells to become more active against the tumor. At the same time, IFN induces greater expression of antigens on the tumor cells, thereby making them more recognizable by the effector cells that have been stimulated.

Antibodies released by B cells bind to antigens on the surface of the tumor cells. Macrophages that recognize antigen-antibody complexes then attack and destroy these cells. They are further stimulated in this activity by IFNγ. Moreover, they may be aided in their destruction of tumor cells by the blood complement system, which will lyse cells that bind antigen-antibody complexes.

The activity of stimulated T and B cells may be inhibited by suppressor T lymphocytes, which are activated in the overall immune response process. In addition, macrophages and tumor cells themselves may produce substances such as prostaglandins, which may further inhibit and, in effect, regulate the extent of immune response activity.

Cytotoxic T lymphocytes are restricted in their responsiveness by the major histocompatibility complexes. In contrast, NK cells and lymphokine-activated T killer cells (LAK) are nonspecific and are not restricted in their activity by the major histocompatibility complex.

Taken together, the immune response in cancer appears to comprise a complex set of interactions between cells and chemical substances that can ultimately either generate an effective action against cells that express particular antigens or inhibit such actions.

Considerations in the Immune Response in Cancer

There are certain assumptions that underlie the hypothesis of a role for the immune response in cancer. The first is that tumor-associated antigens exist. The second is that immunosurveillance, based upon the development of such antigens in association with neoplastic transformation, takes place. The third is that effective coordination between immune recognition, immune activation, immune expression, and neoantigen expression occurs. Unfortunately, each of these assumptions has thus far eluded definitive experimental proof.

Although it has been assumed that tumor-specific, cell-surface antigens exist, what has actually been found is a low prevalence of reactive cell-surface antigens. Some have suggested the nonexpression or low expression of tumor antigens or the masking of such antigens by other molecules to account for this. However, attempts to unmask these antigens or to increase their expression have been unsuccessful in demonstrating the existence of tumor-specific antigens.

Similarly, the theory of immunosurveillance has remained controversial. Theoretically, immunosurveillance may fail because of an absence or a weakness of tumor antigens, lack of immunorecognition, lack of an immune-effector response, or suppression of the immune response. Moreover, even if immunosurveillance is invoked as a cause of occult "spontaneous" regression, the theory seems incompatible with the concept that clinically manifest cancers are antigenic. Indeed, clinically manifest tumors that have escaped surveillance would have had to be functionally nonantigenic. This in turn would obviate the possibility that these tumor cells could stimulate an immune response that might control cancer progression. These thoughts were encapsulated in a review of this topic by Hewitt in 1983: "I do not see how any new strategy for immunotherapy can be conjured out of monoclonal antibodies or the adoptive transfer of specific immune cells when the discriminating specificity of the target cells against which these agents are to act can no longer be asserted."

In evaluating the possible role of the immune response in neoplasia in humans, we are faced with a number of conditions that are difficult to reconcile. Identification of tumor-associated antigens in other than virus-induced tumors remains unproven. The intricacy and complexity of manipulable mechanisms of the immune response make their control and identification difficult. The significance of in vitro assays as a reflection of in vivo events is unclear. Even if we assume that some of the mechanisms involved in the immune response (based on animal experiments and in vitro assays) are active or may be recruited in the clinical setting, we still lack an understanding as to which mechanisms may be important in a particular tumor and at a certain tumor stage. Thus, the role of the immune response in the clinical setting remains problematic.

Tumor Biology and the Immune Response

Events that lead to the generation of cancer are still poorly understood. They are thought to involve the cellular changes that occur as the result of exposure to so-called initiating and promoting factors. The former imply irreversible changes in cellular DNA, while the latter imply proliferation of normal or transformed cells with changes that may be entirely reversible. The discovery of oncogenes and the concomitant possibility that uncontrolled proliferation of cells might reflect either enhanced expression of oncogenes or loss of the controlling influence of anti-oncogenes provided a molecular basis for these events. The mechanisms that induce and account for the development of a cancer, however, are still unclear.

Once a cancer cell has been generated, it takes approximately 20 doublings to produce the 10^6 cells which will occupy a mass of $1\,mm^3$; 27 doublings are required before 10^8 cells are produced, generating a $0.5\text{-}cm^3$ mass which is the size that can first be visualized on X-ray; 30 doublings are required to generate 10^9 cells and the $1\text{-}cm^3$ palpable tumor mass.

By the time of cancer diagnosis in the majority of patients metastases may already have occurred. The cells populating the primary tumor and its metastases may be heterogeneous and express different antigens on their surface. They may also have a variety of other distinguishing heterogeneous phenotypic characteristics. Moreover, zonal differences within the tumor at either primary or secondary sites may include morphology, antigenic properties, sensitivity to cytotoxic drugs, metastatic properties, enzyme capabilities, cell surface receptors, and growth rates.

All of these may influence the capability of the immune response both to detect and effectively control cancer cells in humans. Tumor cell expression of surface antigens, heterogeneity of expression, variation in accessibility to therapeutic agents, ability to escape immunosurveillance, susceptibility to various immune response effector mechanisms, and ability to abrogate these may, individually and in aggregate undermine the potentially effective (based on experimental observations) immune response.

Immunotherapy in Cancer in Humans

The two signal observations that provided the basis of clinical immunotherapy were Coley's recognition in 1900 of the apparent ability of bacterial toxins to stimulate resistance in humans to tumors and Gross' observation in 1950 of tumor-specific transplantation antigens in chemically induced murine tumors. These paved the way for the variety of animal studies and human studies that demonstrated a complexity of immune response mechanisms in tumor systems in both animal models and humans.

As we enter the last decade of the 20th century, however, the efficacy of human cancer immunotherapy remains unproven. That the immune response may play a role in human cancer has been suggested by case reports of presumed spontaneous "remissions," by observations of recurrent tumor growth in patients who have had immunosuppressive therapy, and by an increased incidence of tumors in immunosuppressed patients. In addition, there have been suggestions that the increased cancer risk seen in advanced age may be associated with "immunosenescence" or deterioration of immune response capabilities. This may then be compounded by the developing cancer, which further suppresses immune response capabilities.

The lack of knowledge as to which immune response mechanisms might be active or recruited in the clinical setting and their specificity against the variety of tumors seen, the heterogeneity of cells within both primary and secondary cancer sites, and the failure to identify and utilize tumor antigens in generating and delivering specificity in response enhancement and therapy, have each and in aggregate led to skepticism as to the eventual success of this treatment approach. On the other hand, studies in experimental models, anecdotal observations of tumor regression in humans, and clinical trials in which occasional measureable responses in association with immune response manipulation, have perpetuated enthusiasm in support of additional investigations and optimism that immunotherapy will ultimately have a role in cancer treatment.

Study Design for Immunotherapy in Human Cancer

Notwithstanding the complexity and controversies surrounding the role of immunotherapy in the treatment of human cancer, it is important as well to understand how the unique features of the immune response mandate a particular approach in the design of studies of immunotherapeutic agents in the treatment of human cancers. Particular considerations include an identification of the maximum tolerated dose versus the maximally effective biologic dose, the time course of treatment, the means of delivering the particular agent to the host and to both primary and secondary tumor sites, the question of whether competitive immune response mechanisms might also be recruited, the problem of tumor polyclonality and heterogeneity in designing specific immunotherapeutic approaches against all of the cancer cells, the problem of mixed expression to tumor antigens, and the question of individual immune response capabilities of patients as these may influence the efficacy of the immunotherapeutic approach chosen. Within the context of these considerations, moreover, are found the need to measure the pharmacokinetics of any cellular or humoral agents used for treatment, the need to assay the activity of the biologic responses that may be induced, and the need to correlate biologic responses with in vivo effects on the tumor being treated.

Questions that continue to be of concern in cancer immunotherapy in the clinical setting include whether human cancers contain specific cell-surface antigens that can be recognized and can guide the immune therapeutic approach that is mobilized, whether immunogenic animal tumors are clinically relevant models for human cancers, what the particular roles of cellular versus humoral tumor-specific immunity are in the clinical setting, whether the tumor burden creates a limitation for immunotherapy, whether nonspecific cytotoxicity is relevant in tumor rejection, and whether tumor-specific suppressor cells are potential impediments to successful and effective immunotherapeutic approaches.

In addition, the complexity of immune response mechanisms and their interactions must be considered in attempts to enhance any one of these mechanisms. The response of the tumor in modifying or abrogating host defense mechanisms may also be important in gauging the effects of immunotherapy. Variable antigenicity and biologic behavior of different tumors and their effects in different patients may also influence immunotherapeutic efficacy. The same may be true of immunologic reactivity in different patients, which may be highly variable.

Clinical trials must take each of these considerations into account in their design, treatment assessment, and interpretation of results. The complexity of immunotherapeutic trials because of these considerations is far greater than that of chemotherapeutic trials. Corresponding circumspection and caution in the implementation of such trials and assessment of results are therefore appropriate.

Conclusions

In considering the variety of approaches in immunotherapy that have been used in the management of genitourinary neoplasia, it is highly important to consider the complexity of immune responses that are possible, how their interactions may amplify this complexity, and how difficult it may be to identify one component of this response, enhance its activity, recruit this activity in attacking a cancer, accomplish this with minimal toxicity to the patient, and avoid the stimulation of competitive or inhibitory mechanisms. In the absence of definitive knowledge as to which mechanisms are likely to be effective in treating a particular malignancy, the means by which the immune response can be successfully harnessed continues to require additional study and reassessment of results. It is within this context that we can begin to consider the results of the variety of attempts that have been used to treat genitourinary malignancies by immune response modalities.

Murine Renal Cancer (Renca) Model: Background and Preclinical Studies

R.H. Wiltrout[1], R.L.Hornung[2], H.Futami[1*], T.T. Back[2], H.A. Young[1], and T.J. Sayers[2]

Introduction

About 20 000 new cases of renal cell cancer are diagnosed each year in the USA [1]. Renal cell cancer is relatively resistant to most chemotherapeutic drugs, which makes it a candidate for alternative treatment approaches such as immunotherapy in combination with chemotherapy. The rationale for believing that such an approach may prove useful is based on the fact that primary renal cancers are often fairly vascularized, and responses to biological response modifiers (BRM) such as interferon α (IFNα) and interleukin-2 (IL-2) have been documented [1–4]. These observations suggest that preclinical animal models for renal cancer could be useful for testing the ability of BRM alone, or in combination with chemotherapeutic drugs or other BRM, to mediate antitumor responses.

Several animal models for renal cancer have been described. These models include the Renca adenocarcinoma of BALB/c mice [5], the rat kidney carcinoma (RKC) tumor in the Wistar-Lewis rat [6], and human tumor xenograft models in athymic mice [7, 8]. The model chosen for preclinical study in our laboratory was the Renca adenocarcinoma of BALB/c mice. The Renca tumor arose spontaneously and was originally isolated by Dr. Sarah Stewart at the National Cancer Institute, Bethesda, MD. Subsequently, Murphy and Hrushesky [5] extensively characterized the growth and progression of this tumor in syngeneic mice. They observed progressive growth of Renca in most mice following transfer of as few as 50 viable Renca cells. The tumor spontaneously metastasizes from an intrarenal (IR) implant to the regional lymph nodes, lungs, liver, and spleen, as well as some other organs. The immunogenicity of Renca has been determined to be relatively low [9], although some protection to rechallenge with viable Renca cells following immunization with a membrane vaccine preparation has been reported [10]. In our hands the Renca tumor behaved as reported previously, with progressive metastases

* Dr. H. Futami was supported during the performance of these studies by a Japanese Overseas Cancer Fellowship from the foundation for the Promotion of Cancer Research

[1] Laboratory of Experimental Immunology, Biological Response Modifiers Program, Division of Cancer Treatment, National Cancer Institute, Frederick Cancer Research Facility, Frederick, MD 21701, USA

[2] Biological Carcinogenesis Development Program, Program Resources, Inc., Frederick, MD 21701, USA

F.M.J. Debruyne et al. (Eds.)
Immunotherapy of Renal Cell Carcinoma

viable tumor cells under the capsule of the left kidney [11]. Tumor-bearing mice routinely die between 35 and 45 days.

The studies described herein outline some of the various experimental approaches being pursued in our laboratory with regard to the use of cytokines for preclinical cancer treatment.

Results and Discussion

Adoptive Chemoimmunotherapy of Renca

Initially we found that adoptively transferred lymphokine-activated killer (LAK) cells and exogenously administered recombinant IL-2 (rIL2) synergized with doxorubicin hydrochloride (DOX) for the treatment of Renca. Successful adoptive chemoimmunotherapy (ACIT) of localized intrarenal or intraperitoneal Renca required the administration of rIL2-activated lymphocytes, at least 10 000 U/day for 3–4 days of rIL2, and doses of DOX $\geq$ 4 mg/kg (12–15) which had to be administered prior to the adoptive immunotherapy (AIT). Under these conditions, 60%–90% of mice bearing localized Renca tumors could be rendered disease-free (Table 1) [12, 13]. However, successful treatment of disseminated disease (e.g., that which correlated with clinical stage II, III, or IV) was more complex, requiring nephrectomy of the tumor-bearing kidney and bicompartmental (i.v. + i.p.) administration of both DOX and AIT. By this approach 60%–80% of mice bearing established Renca could be cured of their disease [14].

Table 1. Adoptive chemoimmunotherapy (ACIT) of localized and disseminated Renca

Tumor stage	Treatment approach: Nephrectomy	Treatment approach: Administration of ACIT	% Disease-free survivors	Reference
Localized	No	Local	60–90	[12, 13]
Disseminated	Yes	Bicompartmental	60–80	[14, 15]

BALB/c mice were injected with 1×10^5 viable Renca cells under the capsule of the left kidney. Tumor-bearing mice were treated at various periods of time after Renca injection by a regimen that included 8 mg/kg DOX followed for 3 successive days with the adoptive transfer of 3×10^7 lymphokine-activated killer cells/day plus 10 000 U/rIL2 (generously supplied by Cetus Corporation, Emeryville, CA) per day. In mice with disseminated disease, nephrectomy of the tumor-bearing kidney was performed several hours prior to the initiation of therapy with DOX. For mice bearing early localized tumors, AIT and rIL2 were administered either i.v. or i.p depending on the site of localized tumor growth. Mice bearing disseminated tumors were treated with AIT plus rIL2 administered bicompartmentally (i.v. + i.p.) to assure delivery of therapy to all tumor sites

Distribution and Localization of Adoptively Transferred LAK Effector Cells

Previous studies have reported that bulk LAK cells or adherence-enriched (LAK cells exhibit very limited migratory potential after i.v. injection [16, 17]. However, little is known about the degree of localization of LAK effector cells into tumor sites, and less is known about the distribution capabilities of that fraction of LAK effector cells which is in the process of active proliferation. Therefore, studies were initiated to determine whether LAK effector cells actually distribute widely and localize into tumors following i.v. injection. LAK cells were obtained after 3 days of culture with IL-2 and layered onto a four-layer Percoll density gradient. Virtually all of the cells obtained from the low density (45% Percoll) fraction 2 (Fr2) were large lymphoblasts with large granular lymphocyte (LGL) morphology. The cells obtained from the high density fraction (67% Percoll) were smaller lymphocytes. Approximately 50% of the cells originally layered onto the gradient are recovered from Fr2, and these cells contain > 95% of the total LAK activity of the bulk culture, while the cells obtained from Fr3 and Fr4 contain virtually no LAK activity (Fig. 1). Most of the cells obtained from Fr2 are large lymphoblasts, of which about 25% are actively proliferating [18]. The enriched LAK effector cells were then used to assess their ability to distribute in tumor-bearing mice. The results showed that the enriched LAK effector cells obtained from Fr2 localized poorly to tumor, and most of the actively proliferating cells were no longer detectable after 24 h [18].

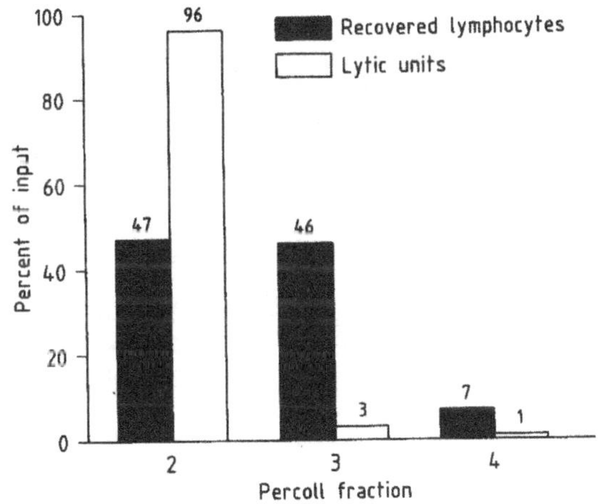

Fig. 1. Enrichment for LAK effector cells by Percoll density fractionation. Splenic lymphocytes were obtained from C57BL/6 mice, cultured with rIL2, and fractionated on Percoll density gradients as in materials and methods. Data presented are from one representative experiment

Treatment of Renca By Flavone Acetic Acid plus rIL2

Because adoptively transferred LAK cells localize poorly into tumors [18], we speculated that cytokines produced by rIL2-activated LAK cells could contribute directly or indirectly to the therapeutic effects of AIT. This hypothesis stimulated studies of other cytokine inducers in combination with rIL2. Subsequently, we found that the synthetic investigational drug flavone acetic acid (FAA) with rIL2 was effective in the therapy of Renca. FAA has shown to augment systemic NK activity potently (as assessed in the peripheral blood, spleen, lungs, and liver) and to synergize with rIL2 for the successful treatment of advanced Renca (40%–90% long-term, disease-free survivors [19]). Cytokines induced by FAA have been implicated in its therapeutic synergy with rIL2. Northern blot analysis of spleen cells for FAA-treated mice revealed the induction, in a dose- and time-dependent manner, of mRNA, and bioassays showed the production of biologically active proteins for tumor necrosis factor α (TNFα), IFNα, and IFNγ from splenic or hepatic leukocytes [20, 21]. Doses of FAA active for cytokine induction correlated well with therapeutic synergy with rIL2 (Table 2). These observations led to further studies in which IFNα and IFNγ were shown to have enhanced antitumor effects in vitro and in vivo against localized Renca [22]. Subsequent experiments have shown that the administration of IFNα, IFNγ, and TNFα, in the same order as that in which the genes are induced by FAA, in conjunction with IL-2 is able to cure some mice bearing disseminated Renca (Wiltrout et al., manuscript in preparation).

Table 2. Dose-dependent cytokine gene expression and therapeutic synergy with rIL2

Dose of FAA (mg/kg)	Induction of mRNA[a]			Survival of Renca-bearing mice following treatment with FAA + rIL2 (%)[b]
	TNFα	IFNγ	IFNα	
0	–	–	–	0
100	–	–	–	0– 10
150	++	++	++	20– 50
200	++++	++++	++++	40–100

FAA, flavone acetic acid

[a] BALB/c mice were treated with various doses of FAA and cytokine gene expression assessed by Northern blot analysis of mRNA derived from spleen cells 2 h after FAA administration. Intensity of hybridization is presented on a scale of + → ++++

[b] BALB/c mice were injected under the capsule of the left kidney with 1×10^5 viable Renca cells 11 days prior to the administration of different doses of FAA plus 10 000 U/day rIL2. The mice were then monitored for survival for at least 100 days. Data presented are a summary of three separate experiments

Table 3. Effects of alkalinization on biologic response modification and therapeutic efficacy of FAA

Parameter	Decrease %
Induction of mRNA for IFNα and IFNγ	>90
Induction of mRNA for TNFα	>50
Production of serum IFN activity	>75
Augmentation of splenic or hepatic natural killer activity	40–60
Therapeutic synergy with rIL2	40–90

Alkalinization of mice was performed by injecting 0.5 ml of 5% $NaHCO_3$ i.p. 1 h prior to the administration of FAA. This procedure raised the urine pH from about 5.8 to 7.8. Data presented were derived from 5 separate experiments

Effect of In Vivo Alkalinization on the Therapeutic and Immunomodulatory Effects of FAA

A further implication for the role of induced cytokines in the antitumor effects of FAA plus rIL2 derives from more recent studies performed in alkalinized mice [23]. The effect of alkalinization on FAA plus rIL2 therapy was investigated because clinical trials of FAA alone demonstrated little therapeutic efficacy, although some immune modulation in the form of increased NK and serum IFN activity has been reported [24]. Interestingly, in most studies patients were alkalinized to prevent the crystallization of FAA in the renal tubules. Thus, we performed studies to determine the effects of alkalinization on FAA-induced cytokine induction and therapeutic synergy with rIL2 in Renca-bearing mice (Table 3). The results showed that the upregulation of mRNA for TNFα, IFNγ, and IFNα by FAA was dramatically reduced or completely eliminated in alkalinized mice. Further, FAA plus rIL2 was therapeutically ineffective (3% long-term survivors) in alkalinized Renca-bearing mice when compared with nonalkalinized controls (42% long-term survivors). The possible mechanism for this observation could relate to an accelerated clearance of FAA in alkalinized mice or patients or to an alteration in the degradation products that may be the active immunomodulatory or immunotherapeutic moieties.

Conclusions

Overall, our results to date demonstrate that immunotherapeutic approaches that incorporate rIL2 and chemotherapy can yield improved therapeutic effects against Renca. The data suggest that the contributions of LAK cells and FAA to the antitumor effects of LAK plus rIL2 or FAA plus rIL2 therapies may be mediated through cytokines produced by LAK cells or induced by FAA. The correlation between cytokine induction and therapeutic effects is particularly striking since LAK effector cells produce considerable amounts of several cytokines yet do not localize well into tumors. Conversely, doses of FAA that do not induce cytokines also do not demonstrate therapeutic synergy with rIL2. These results suggest that the antitumor effects of rIL2 can be markedly enhanced by its use in combination with other cytokines. The mechanisms for these enhanced antitumor effects could include direct antiproliferative effects of cytokines as well as cytokine-induced immune modulation. Considerably more research will be required to identify optimized regimens for the administration of multiple cytokines and to understand the contribution of the various mechanisms to the observed antitumor effects.

References

1. Bassil B, Dosoretz DE, Prout GR Jr (1985) Validation of the tumor, nodes, and metastasis classification of renal cell carcinoma. J Urol 134:450–454
2. Clark JW, Longo DL (1987) Interferons in cancer therapy. In: DeVita VT Jr, Hellman S, Rosenberg SA (eds) Cancer: Principles and practice of oncology, vol 1, pp 1–15
3. Buzaid AC, Robertone A, Kisala C, Salmon SE (1987) Phase II study of interferon Alfa-2a, recombinant (Roferon-A) in metastatic renal cell carcinoma. J Clin Oncol 5:1083–1089
4. Rosenberg SA (1989) Clinical immunotherapy studies in the surgery branch of U.S. National Cancer Institute: Brief review. Can Treat Rev 16 [Suppl A]:115–121
5. Murphy GP, Hrushesky WJ (1973) A murine renal cell carcinoma. J Natl Cancer Inst 50:1013–1025
6. deVere White R, Olsson CA (1980) Renal adenocarcinoma in the rat: A new tumor model. Investigative Urol 17:405–411
7. Kozlowski JM, Fidler IJ, Campbell D, Xu Z, Kaighn ME, Hart IR (1984) Metastatic behavior of human tumor cell lines grown in the nude mouse. Cancer Res 44:3522–3529
8. Naito S, Giavazzi R, Walker SM, Itoh K, Mayo J, Fidler IJ (1987) Growth and metastatic behavior of human tumor cells implanted into nude and beige nude mice. Clin Exp Metastasis 5:135–146
9. Hrushesky WJ, Murphy GP (1973) Investigation of a new renal tumor model. J Surg Res 15:327–332
10. Huben RP, Connelly R, Goldrosen MH, Murphy GP, Pontes JE (1983) Immunotherapy of a murine renal cancer. J Urol 129:1075–1078
11. Salup R, Herberman RB, Wiltrout RH (1985) Role of natural killer activity in development of spontaneous metastases in murine renal cancer. J Urol 134:1236–1241
12. Salup RR, Wiltrout RH (1986) Treatment of adenocarcinoma in the peritoneum of mice: Chemoimmunotherapy with IL-2 stimulated cytotoxic lymphocytes as a model for treatment of minimal residual disease. Cancer Immunol Immunother 22:31–36
13. Salup RR, Wiltrout RH (1986) Adjuvant immunotherapy of established murine renal cancer by interleukin 2-stimulated cytotoxic lymphocytes. Cancer Res 46:3358–3363
14. Salup RR, Back TA, Wiltrout RH (1987) Successful treatment of advanced murine renal cell cancer by bicompartmental adoptive chemoimmunotherapy. J Immunol 138:641–647
15. Wiltrout RH, Salup RR (1988) Adoptive immunotherapy in combination with chemotherapy for cancer treatment. Prog Exp Tumor Res 32:128–153
16. Maghazachi AA, Goldfarb RH, Herberman RB (1988) Influence of T cells on the expression of lymphokine-activated killer cell activity and in vivo tissue distribution. J Immunol 141:4039–4046

17. Maghazachi AA, Herberman RB, Vujanovic NL, Hiserodt JC (1988) In vivo distribution and tissue localization of highly purified rat lymphokine-activated killer (LAK) cells. Cell Immunol 115:179–194
18. Futami H, Pilaro AM, Gruys ME, Back TT, Young HA, Wiltrout RH (1990) In vivo distribution and cytokine gene expression by enriched mouse LAK effector cells. Biotherapy (in press)
19. Wiltrout RH, Boyd MR, Back TC, Salup RR, Arthur JA, Hornung RL (1988) Flavone-8-acetic acid augments systemic natural killer cell activity and synergizes with interleukin 2 for treatment of murine renal cancer. J Immunol 140:3261–3265
20. Hornung RL, Back TC, Zaharko DS, Urba WJ, Longo DL, Wiltrout RH (1988) Augmentation of natural killer (NK) activity, induction of interferon and development of tumor immunity during the successful treatment of established murine renal cancer using flavone acetic acid (FAA) and interleukin 2. J Immunol 141:3671–3679
21. Mace KF, Hornung RC, Wiltrout RH, Young HA (1990) Induction of cytokine gene expression in vivo by flavone acetic acid: Strict dose dependency and correlation with therapeutic efficacy against murine renal cancer. Cancer Res 50:1742–1747
22. Sayers TJ, Wiltrout TA, McCormick K, Husted C, Wiltrout RH (1990) Antitumor effects of IFNα and IFNγ on a murine renal cancer (Renca) in vitro and in vivo. Cancer Res 50:5414–5420
23. Futami H, Hornung RL, Back TT, Gruys ME, Wiltrout RH (1990) Effect of systemic alkalinization on biologic response modification and therapeutic antitumor efficacy of flavone acetic acid plus recombinant interleukin 2. Cancer Res (in press)
24. Urba WJ, Longo DL, Lombardo FA, Weiss RB (1988) Enhancement of natural killer activity in human peripheral blood by flavone acetic acid. J Natl Cancer Inst 80:521–525

Renal Cell Carcinoma: Experimental Metastases

J. J. Killion and I. J. Fidler[1]

Introduction

During the past 2 decades, our understanding of the pathogenesis of metastasis has increased considerably, yet improvements in the treatment of metastatic disease produced by the common tumors of humans have been relatively limited. Although there is no question that major advances in general patient care, surgical resection of neoplasms, and adjuvant therapies have occurred, the majority of deaths from cancer are still caused by metastases that are resistant to therapy [1–3]. The major barrier to the eradication of metastases is that the cancer cells in both primary tumors and in metastases are biologically heterogeneous. This heterogeneity is manifested in a wide range of cell properties, such as cell surface enzymes, receptors, karyotypes, morphology, growth properties, and ability to invade and produce metastasis. Of particular significance to oncologists, neoplasms display a heterogeneous response to a variety of therapeutic agents. Because biological heterogeneity occurs among cancers of different histologic origins (e.g., renal v. breast cancer), among tumors of the same histologic origin but in different patients (intertumoral heterogeneity), and within a single neoplasm (intratumoral heterogeneity), continual empiricism in the treatment of cancer is unlikely to produce significant improvement. Stated differently, new therapeutic modalities for cancer metastasis must be based on answers to the questions of how biological heterogeneity is regulated in neoplasms and what processes generate metastasis [3–5].

The concept that neoplasms are heterogeneous and contain cells with different biological properties is not new. Some 100 years ago, the British surgeon Stephen Paget analyzed autopsies of over 700 patients with breast cancer and concluded that the nonrandom pattern of metastasis was not due to chance. Rather, metastases resulted from the proliferation of a few tumor cells (the seed) in the favorable milieu provided by some organs (the soil). A current definition of Paget's hypothesis consists of three principles. First, as stated above, neoplasms are heterogeneous for metastatic properties. Second, the process of metastasis is sequential and selective and contains stochastic elements. Third, the production of clinical metastases is dependent upon the interaction of metastatic cells with various host factors. We shall describe the general properties of the tumor-host relationship that allow the

[1] Department of Cell Biology, The University of Texas M.D., Anderson Cancer Center, 1515 Holcombe Boulevard, Houston, Texas 77030, USA

F.M.J. Debruyne et al. (Eds.)
Immunotherapy of Renal Cell Carcinoma

emergence of metastatic tumor populations and, more specifically, data from our laboratory on the metastatic properties of human renal cell carcinoma (HRCC) in athymic (nude) mice. Development of this model may lead to an ability to evaluate potential therapeutic modalities against renal cancer.

The Pathogenesis of Metastases

The process of cancer metastatasis consists of a series of sequential, interlinked steps [6, 7]. To produce a clinically relevant metastasis, a tumor cell must complete a series of potentially lethal interactions with various host factors. Metastasis begins with the growth of tumor cells and invasion into host stroma surrounding the primary neoplasm. Tumor cell invasion into blood vessels and lymphatics is facilitated by the production of enzymes such as cathepsin B and plasminogen activator and various collagenases that can lyse basement membranes and host connective tissues. During local invasion and subsequent to the arrest and attachment of metastatic cells in distant capillary beds, the tumor cells must penetrate the basement membranes that surround the blood vessels. Basement membranes and connective tissues consist of collagens, elastin, glycoproteins, and various proteoglycans. The proportion of these varies among basement membranes of different tissues. Dissolution of the basement membrane has been observed in areas of tumor invasion, and favored sites of tumor cell attachment and destruction are the collagen and proteoglycan components. Metastatic tumor cells show preferential attachment to type IV collagen, and these cells may secrete collagenase.

During invasion, tumor cells can easily penetrate small lymphatic vessels and be passively transported in the lymph to lymph nodes, where numerous lymphatic venous communications are found. Hence, tumor cells have the capability of reaching the general circulation, as well as regional areas near their site of origin. During blood-borne metastasis, tumor cells must survive transport in the circulation, adhere to small blood vessels at distant capillary beds, and there invade the vessel wall.

Because the vast majority of circulating cells do not survive, the mere presence of tumor cells in the bloodstream does not itself constitute metastasis. By using radiolabeled tumor cells, it was found that 24 h after entry into the circulation less than 1% of the cells were viable. Less than 0.1% eventually survived to form metastases [3]. Parameters of successful metastases included the number of cells in the circulation and the formation of multicell emboli consisting of only tumor cells or tumor and host cells.

The subsequent interactions of metastatic cells with cells of the vascular endothelium include nonspecific lodgement of cell emboli and the formation of stable adhesions between tumor cells and small-vessel endothelial cells. Increased coagulation of the blood in some cancer patients may aid in the formation of metastases. Extravasation of arrested tumor cells is believed to operate by mechanisms similar to those responsible for local invasion. Subsequent to arrest, tumor cells grow and destroy the surrounding vessel, penetrate the endothelial basement membrane, or follow migrating white blood cells. The ability of malignant cells to extravasate into surrounding tissues may be, in part, due to selective adherence to endothelial cells.

The survival, invasion, and growth of malignant cells at particular secondary sites also involve their response to tissue and organ factors. Tumor cells recognize tissue-specific motility factors, and they may respond to organ-specific factors that influence their growth. Surviving metastatic cells may also produce their own growth factors (autocrine stimulation), which allows them to establish autonomy from their immediate microenvironment. When one considers the multitude of events that metastatic tumor cells must be able to survive, metastases may appear to be due to the random survival of a few cells. However, the data show that the process of metastasis does contain stochastic elements and that secondary growths result from the survival of unique subpopulations of tumor cells [3, 7].

Use of the Athymic Mouse Model for Studies of Human Metastases

Studies in animals have shown that metastases can arise from the nonrandom spread of specialized subpopulations of cells that preexist within the primary tumor. In addition, metastases can be clonal in their origin, and different metastatic lesions can originate from different progenitor cells. Similar studies on the metastatic properties of human tumors require models in which the in vivo growth of human tumors is assessed in nude mice [8]. Most human tumors transplanted into nude mice by the intravenous (i.v.), intraperitoneal (i.p.), subcutaneous (s.c.), or intramuscular routes rarely produce metastasis, regardless of their clinical behavior in patients. This may be related to parameters associated with the housing of the nude mice, i.e., they must be specific pathogen-free and have low levels of spontaneous macrophage activity. In addition, the composition and pH of the drinking water, the lighting cycle of the animal facility, and the type of cage bedding used may indirectly affect the in vivo growth of human tumors. Of most importance is the observation that the metastatic behavior of tumors depends upon the site of their implantation, suggesting that both intrinsic properties of the metastatic tumor cell and host factors, perhaps organ-specific, determine the metastatic behavior of human neoplasms in nude mice.

Biological Properties of HRCC in Nude Mice

Influence of Implantation Site upon Biological Properties of HRCC. Experiments were designed to determine the influence of implantation site on the growth of local "primary tumors" and the metastatic behavior of HRCC cells [9]. HRCC lines were established in vitro from a surgical specimen (SN12C) or from a liver metastasis produced in BALB/c nude mice by cells from the original specimen implanted into their kidney (SN12L1). Equal numbers of cultured HRCC cells of both lines were injected into the subcutis and under the renal capsule (RSC) of nude mice. Tumor growth and metastatic behavior were monitored. In both cell lines, tumor cells injected into the RSC displayed faster growth and produced more systemic metastases than did cells injected s.c. The kidney tumors were large, invasive, highly vascularized, and nonencapsulated and had minimal central necrosis. In contrast, the subcutaneous tumors were highly encapsulated, with peripheral vascularization and extensive necrosis that developed as early as 2 weeks after s.c. implantation. The SN12L1 cells were also implanted into nude mice by i.v., i.p., and intrasplenic injections. The most dramatic production of metastasis occurred after the tumor cells were injected into the kidney. These results indicate that the biologic behavior of this HRCC is influenced by the implantation site in nude mice. At least for this cell line, the kidney is the natural organ for growth, and implantation into the RSC is advantageous for the study of the biology of HRCC in nude mice.

Influence of Implantation Site upon Karyotypic Properties of HRCC. The parent line SN12C is highly heterogeneous with respect to 34 separate chromosome markers, 4 of which are present in nearly all of the cells. Subcutaneous implantation of SN12C resulted in tumor growth, but karyotypic analysis revealed selection for a homogeneous population of cells and total loss of 3 out of 4 of the dominant markers. Hence, this tumor may not be representative of the parent tumor population. However, implantation of the parent cell line SN12C into the renal subcapsule and isolation of a liver metastasis from mice bearing kidney-implanted tumor allowed us to demonstrate that the karyotype of these cell lines closely resembled that of the parental tumor, although new markers also appeared.

Evidence for Metastatic Heterogeneity of HRCC. HRCC SN12C is heterogeneous and contains cells with different metastatic properties [10]. Clonal populations of SN12C cells were isolated by a double-dilution technique. Cells from parental and 11 clonal lines were injected s.c., i.v., and into the RSC of nude mice. Seven cloned lines differed significantly from the parent line in their ability to produce pulmonary metastases after RSC implantation. These results indicate that this HRCC is heterogeneous for metastasis, and this heterogeneity can be demonstrated using the proper site of tumor implantation.

In Vivo Selection of Highly Metastatic Cells of SN12 HRCC. Orthotopic implantation of HRCC cells into nude mice will produce distant metastases, thus allowing for the selection of variant cells with high metastatic potential [11]. The RSC of adult nude mice was injected with SN12C cells; the mice were killed when they became moribund. Cell lines were established from either single or multiple HRCC lung metastases. The i.v. injection of many (but not all) of the metastasis-derived lines produced significantly more experimental metastases than did the parental cells. The injection of cells into the RSC demonstrated that, in general, cells derived from spontaneous metastases were more metastatic than cells of the parental line. Hence, adult nude mice can be used to select HRCC cells with high metastatic potential.

Influence of Organ-Specific Factors on the Growth of SN12 HRCC

It has been reported that nephrectomy of tumor-bearing, conventional mice may result in the stimulation of tumor growth, presumably due to the presence of circulating renotropic factors that lead to compensatory hypertrophy in the contralateral kidney [12, 13]. Preliminary studies in our laboratory indicate that the development of lung metastases and the rate of DNA synthesis of HRCC cells may be influenced by nephrectomy of tumor-bearing nude mice. Mice were injected i.v. with SN12pm6 cells (derived from a pulmonary metastasis), and nephrectomy was performed 3 weeks later. Autopsy of the mice revealed an increase in the number of lung colonies in the nephrectomized mice compared with those that underwent sham nephrectomy. An increase in the amount of DNA synthesis in s.c. tumors could also be detected in nude mice that were nephrectomized. However, these studies are sensitive to uncharacterized parameters of proper timing of surgery, tumor burden, and anatomical location. Hence, this model of organ-mediated stimulation of tumor cell growth has not yet been fully developed.

References

1. Fidler IJ, Hart IR (1982) Biological diversity in metastatic neoplasms: Origins and implications. Science 217:938–1003
2. Fidler IJ, Poste G (1985) The cellular heterogeneity of malignant neoplasms: Implications for adjuvant chemotherapy. Semin Oncol 12:207–221
3. Fidler IJ, Balch CM (1987) The biology of cancer metastasis and implications for therapy. Curr Probl Surg 24:130–209
4. Nicolson GL (1984) Generation of phenotypic diversity and progression in metastatic tumors. Cancer Metastasis Rev 3:25–42
5. Heppner G (1984) Tumor heterogeneity. Cancer Res 44:2259–2265
6. Poste G, Fidler IJ (1980) The pathogenesis of cancer metastasis. Nature 283:139–146
7. Killion JJ, Fidler IJ (1989) The biology of tumor metastasis. Semin Oncol 16:106–115
8. Fidler IJ (1986) Rationale and methods for the use of nude mice to study the biology and therapy of human cancer metastasis. Cancer Metastasis Reviews 5:29–49
9. Naito S, von Eschenbach AC, Fidler IJ (1987) Different growth patterns and biological behavior of human renal cell carcinoma implanted into different organs of nude mice. J Natl Cancer Inst 78:377–385
10. Naito S, Walker SM, von Eschenbach AC, Fidler IJ (1988) Evidence for metastatic heterogeneity of human renal cell carcinoma. Anticancer Res 8:1163–1168
11. Naito S, Walker SM, Fidler IJ (1989) In vivo selection of human renal cell carcinoma cells with high metastatic potential in nude mice. Clin Exptl Metastasis 7:381–389
12. Pliskin ME, Prehn RT (1975) Stimulation of liver regeneration and compensatory kidney hyperplasia by passive transfer of spleen cells. J Reticuloendothel Soc 17:290–299
13. Murphy GP, Tritsch GL, Sufrin G, Williams PD (1985) Kinetics of formation of renotropic growth factor. Urology 25:622–624

Oncogenes in Renal Cell Carcinoma

E. A. Klein[1]

The study of oncogenes in human tumors has yielded significant insights into the molecular basis for the origin, development, and progression of many cancers and sometimes provided clinically useful information. These were initially cytogenetic characterization and detailed mapping studies which identified the location of oncogenes near chromosomal breakpoints. With advances in molecular technology and applying lessons learned from the study of hematologic tumors, the study of oncogenes in human solid tumors has advanced significantly in the past several years. At present, information regarding which oncogenes are important in renal cell carcinoma (RCC) and detailed study of their structure, expression, modes of action, and biologic significance are limited. This chapter will review the published data on oncogenes in renal cancers and attempt to integrate the findings into models of known oncogene function. Areas in which information is lacking will be highlighted and directions for future studies suggested.

In 1979 Cohen and colleagues described a family in which a constitutional translocation t(3;8)(p21;q24) (Fig. 1A) was associated with renal cell carcinoma [1]. The occurrence of the translocation and tumor exhibited strict concordance. Subsequently, a variety of abnormalities (deletions, insertions, and translocations) involving the region 3p11→3p21 of chromosome 3 has been reported both in familial and sporadic forms of RCC (Fig. 1B), with the common denominator being loss of chromosomal material from 3p [2]. Several molecular oncogene studies of RCC have led on from these cytogenetic observations.

Deregulation of c-*myc*, which is located at 8q24, was suggested by the translocation breakpoint of 8q24 observed in familial RCC (Fig. 1A); one hypothesis was that activation of c-*myc* by translocation, which is important in the genesis of Burkitt's lymphoma, might also be important in RCC. Although c-*myc* is frequently expressed in RCC [3–5], the level of expression appears to be no higher than in normal tissue [3, 6]. Furthermore, recent mapping studies using pulsed-field electrophoresis have shown that the 8q24 break was not within a 1500-kb region surrounding c-*myc* [6]. These observations suggest that c-*myc* activation by translocation or structural changes within the gene is not important in RCC.

Activation by deregulated transcription of the *raf*-1 oncogene was also suggested by cytogenetic observations. Deletions of 3p in sporadic RCC were observed to

[1] Section of Urologic Oncology, Department of Urology, Cleveland Clinic Foundation, 9500 Euclid Avenue, Cleveland, OH 44195, USA

F.M.J. Debruyne et al. (Eds.)
Immunotherapy of Renal Cell Carcinoma

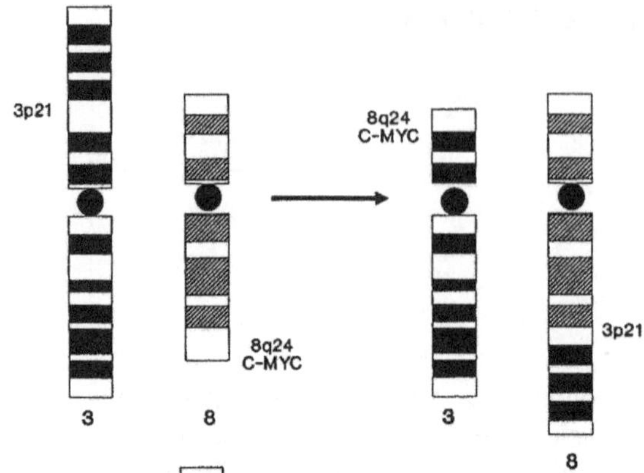

Fig. 1A. Idiogram of translocation between chromosomes 3 and 8 observed in a family with renal cell carcinoma. This translocation resulted in the transposition of the c-myc oncogene to the short arm of chromosome 3

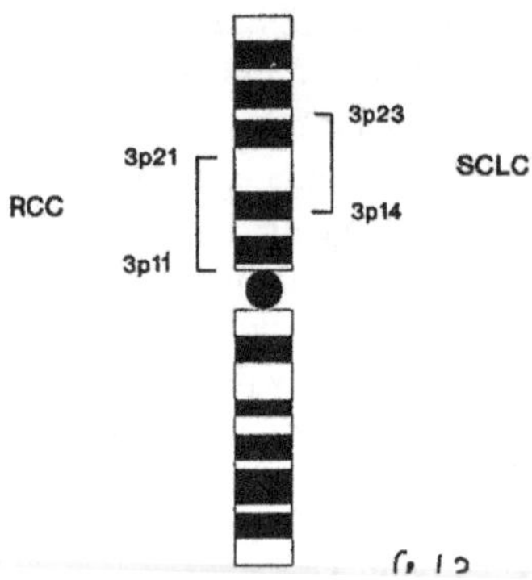

Fig. 1B. Idiogram of chromosome 3 showing areas typically deleted in renal cell carcinoma (RCC) and small cell lung cancer (SCLC)

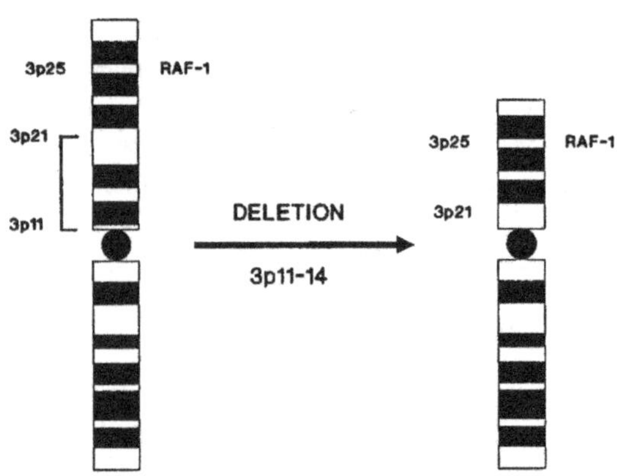

Fig. 1C. Idiogram illustrating proximal shift of the raf 1 oncogene resulting from a deletion of 3p11-14

cause a proximal shift of c-*raf*-1 (located at 3p25) in some tumors (Fig. 1C) [7]. Although c-*raf*-1 expression is observed in RCC, the levels of expression are no higher than in normal tissue [8].

The cytogenetic observations of 3p deletions have been substantiated by the molecular detection of loss of heterozygosity for alleles in this region [9, 10]. Drawing an analogy from the study of retinoblastoma, these data suggest that loss of a tumor-suppressing allele (antioncogene) from 3p may be important in RCC (Fig. 2). This hypothesis suggests that two mutations must occur in the wild-type allele (RCC+ in Fig. 2) for a tumor to occur; the presence of a single normal allele is sufficient to suppress tumorigenesis. In sporadic tumors both mutations (RCC-) are somatic, and tumors occur unifocally and late in life (Fig. 2, top). In familial RCC, as seen in Von Hippel-Lindau disease (VHL), one mutation is inherited in the germline and occurs in all cells of both kidneys (Fig. 2, bottom); consequently, the RCC in VHL tends to be multifocal and bilateral and occurs at an earlier age. Validation of this hypothesis awaits detailed mapping studies of the "least common deleted segment" in order to identify the gene of interest. Such work will also likely identify a tumor suppressor gene important in small cell lung cancer (SCLC) which shares deletion of chromosome 3 with RCC as a characteristic cytogenetic finding (Fig. 1B).

Other investigators have adopted a less direct approach to the identification of oncogenes important in RCC. Slamon identified expression of c-*fes*, c-*fos*, c-*myc*, c-Ha-*ras*, and c-Ki-*ras* in sporadic RCC, although not at levels higher than in adjacent normal kidney; conversely, c-*abl*, c-*myc*, and c-*src* were not expressed in any tumors [3]. Karthaus et al. made similar observations in both primary tumors and nude mice xenografts, although c-*abl* was expressed in most of the xenografts [4, 5]. In addition, these investigators identified a novel 4.5-kb c-*fes* transcript in two

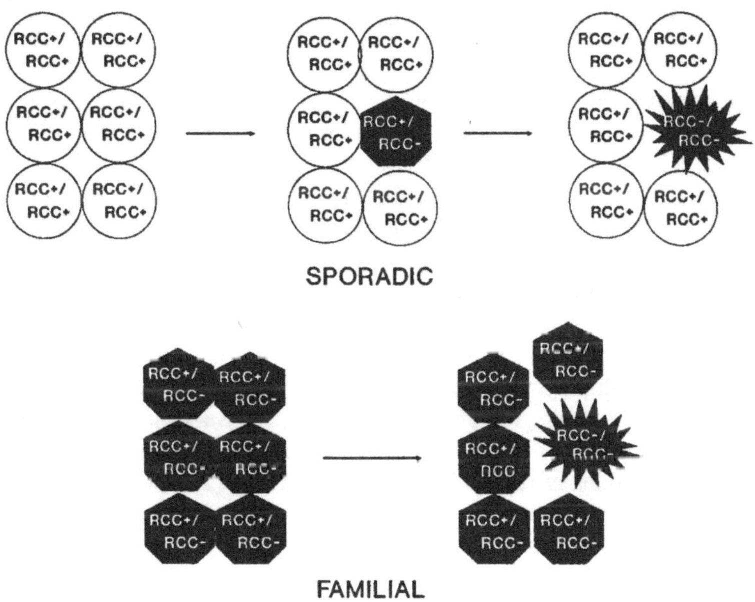

Fig. 2. Schematic representation of loss of a tumor suppressor gene leading to renal cell carcinoma in sporadic RCC. In sporadic RCC 2 somatic mutations of mature renal tissue are necessary for tumor formation. In familial forms of RCC, such as occurs in Von Hippel-Lindau disease, the first mutation is inherited in every renal epithelial cell, putting each cell at risk for tumor formation. Only a single somatic mutation, corresponding to the second mutation in sporadic RCC, is necessary for tumorigenesis. RCC+ = normal tumor suppressor gene; RCC- = inactivated or deleted suppressor gene

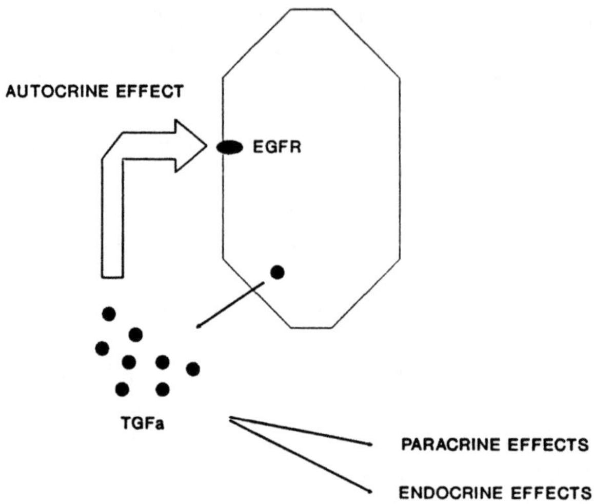

Fig. 3. Schematic diagram illustrating the hypothesized autocrine effect of transforming growth factor alpha in RCC. A renal epithelial cell synthesizes transforming growth factor alpha which may have effects on adjacent cells (paracrine effects), distant cells (endocrine effects), or may stimulate the cell which synthesized it (autocrine effect)

primary RCC, an observation of as yet unknown significance. Several examinations of primary tumors including RCC screened for oncogene amplification have failed to identify significant genomic changes in any of the previously mentioned oncogenes or c-*erb*-B, N-*myc*, or c-*sis* [4, 11].

Detailed study of the *ras* oncogenes has shown a low incidence of activated Ha-*ras* alleles by point mutation. In one reported study, 2 of 16 tumors contained transforming sequences homologous to Ha-*ras* as detected by the NIH/3T3 transfection assay [8]. Protein electrophoretic and Southern blot analysis revealed typical mutations at codons 12 and 61 in these tumors. Half of them showed restriction fragment length polymorphism (RFLP) for a *Bam*HI site in Ha-*ras*; one exhibited loss of heterozygosity for one of the alleles. More recent studies using the more sensitive technique of polymerase chain reaction have confirmed the low incidence of point mutations in *ras* alleles in sporadic RCC [12]. It would appear from these data that *ras* point mutations are probably not important in most RCC.

An autocrine method of RCC growth has recently been hypothesized based on two other observations. Mydlo et al. observed transcription of transforming growth factor alpha (TGFa) in five stage I RCC without detectable levels in normal kidney [13]. The same tumors expressed a threefold higher level of epidermal growth factor receptor (EGFR) gene transcription than in nonneoplastic tissue. Coupled with other observations of EGFR expression in kidney [14, 15] and the known ability of TGFa to bind EGFR, the results suggest a mechanism by which RCC may perpetuate its own growth (Fig. 3).

Finally, few attempts at correlating the clinical behavior of RCC with oncogene structure, amplification, or expression have been reported. One such study demonstrated that 15 of 16 metastatic RCC contained one or another allelic pattern as defined by an RFLP for the L-*myc* oncogene, while 10 of 11 of the tumors with the third pattern were nonmetastatic [16]. There was no correlation of grade or capsular penetration with the RFLPs. The findings are particularly interesting in view of the fact that L-*myc* is expressed in SCLC, suggesting a second common genetic mechanism for RCC and SCLC.

In summary, no unifying hypothesis or model of oncogene structure or function in RCC has emerged to date. The most promising areas of study seem to be the identification of a putative tumor suppressor gene on chromosome 3p, as well as further exploration of the role of growth factor/growth factor receptor genes. Systematic analysis of testable hypotheses rather than shotgun approaches to the detection of oncogene expression or structure is also needed.

References

1. Cohen AJ et al. (1979) Hereditary renal cell carcinoma associated with a chromosomal translocation. N Engl J Med 301:592
2. Carroll PR et al. (1987) Abnormalities of chromosome region 3p12-14 characterize clear cell renal cell carcinoma. Cancer Genet Cytogenet 26:253
3. Slamon DJ et al. (1984) Expression of cellular oncogenes in human malignancies. Science 224:256
4. Karthaus HFM et al. (1987) Expression of proto-oncogenes in xenografts of human renal cell carcinomas. Urol Res 15:349
5. Karthaus HFM et al. (1986) Expression of the human fes cellular oncogene in renal cell tumors. Urol Res 14:123
6. Gemmill RM et al. (1989) A 1.5-megabase restriction map surrounding MYC does not include the translocation breakpoint in familial renal cell carcinoma. Genomics 4:28
7. Teyssier JR (1986) Recurrent deletion of the short arm of chromosome 3 in human renal cell carcinoma: shift of the raf-1 locus. J Natl Cancer Inst 77:6
8. Fujita J et al. (1988) Activated H-ras oncogenes in human kidney tumors. Cancer Res 48:5251
9. Zbar B et al. (1987) Loss of alleles of loci on the short arm of chromosome 3 in renal cell carcinoma. Nature 327:722
10. Kovacs G et al. (1988) Consistent chromosome 3p deletion and loss of heterozygosity in renal cell carcinoma. Proc Natl Acad Sci USA 85:1571
11. Masuda H et al. (1987) Specificity of proto-oncogene amplification in human malignant diseases. Mol Biol Med 4:213
12. Nanus D et al. (1990) Infrequent ras oncogene point mutations in renal cell carcinoma. J Urol 143:175
13. Mydlo JB et al. (1989) Expression of transforming growth factor alpha and epidermal growth factor receptor messenger RNA in neoplastic and nonneoplastic human kidney tissue. Cancer Res 49:3407
14. Lau JLT et al. (1988) Epidermal growth factor in the normal and neoplastic kidney and bladder. J Urol 139:170
15. Singletary SE et al. (1988) Biological effect of epidermal growth factor in the in vitro growth of human tumors. Cancer Res 47:403
16. Kakehi Y, Yoshida O (1989) Restriction fragment length polymorphism of the L-myc gene and susceptibility to metastasis in renal cancer patients. Int J Cancer 43:391

Molecular Basis and Clinical Relevance of MDR1 Gene Expression in Renal Cell Carcinoma

Y. Kakehi and O. Yoshida[1]

Introduction

One of the major problems in cancer chemotherapy is the development of drug resistance during treatment. Such resistance may occur during primary therapy or be acquired during subsequent treatment. Recent progress has been made in the genetic analysis of P-glycoprotein (P170), a 170-kilodalton transmembrane glycoprotein encoded by the MDR1 gene [1]. It has been reported that P170 works as an energy-dependent efflux pump to expel several structurally unrelated agents including *Vinca* alkaloids and anthracyclines from multidrug-resistant cell lines [2]. The MDR1 gene is expressed in various normal human organs such as adrenal, liver, kidney, and colon, and in cancers which originated from these organs [3]. These findings suggest that those tumors in which overexpression of MDR1 occurs can be intrinsically drug resistant. Renal cell carcinoma (RCC) is well known as one of the neoplasms which are naturally quite resistant to chemotherapeutic agents. In this chapter, we discuss the molecular basis and clinical relevance of MDR1 gene expression in RCC.

MDR1 Messenger RNA Levels in Genitourinary Tumors

Immunohistochemical staining using a monoclonal antibody, MRK-16, revealed that in the kidney P170 is located on the brush border of proximal tubular cells [4]. Since most RCCs are considered to be of proximal tubular cell origin, the MDR1 gene is expected to be expressed. Figure 1 shows a slot blot analysis of RNA from RCC tissue samples as well as the adjacent normal kidneys and other genitourinary tumor tissues. In more than one-half of the RCC samples, the MDR1 mRNA levels were increased to be comparable with that of the adjacent normal kidney tissues. On the other hand, all other genitourinary cancer samples (8 urothelial tumors, 2 prostatic cancers, and 3 testis tumors) had low levels of MDR1 mRNA. The Northern blot analysis of RNA extracted from these RCC samples and from normal kidney tissues showed a 4.5 kb mRNA species which corresponds to the size of P170 mRNA [5].

[1] Department of Urology, Kyoto University Faculty of Medicine, Kyoto, Japan

F.M.J. Debruyne et al. (Eds.)
Immunotherapy of Renal Cell Carcinoma

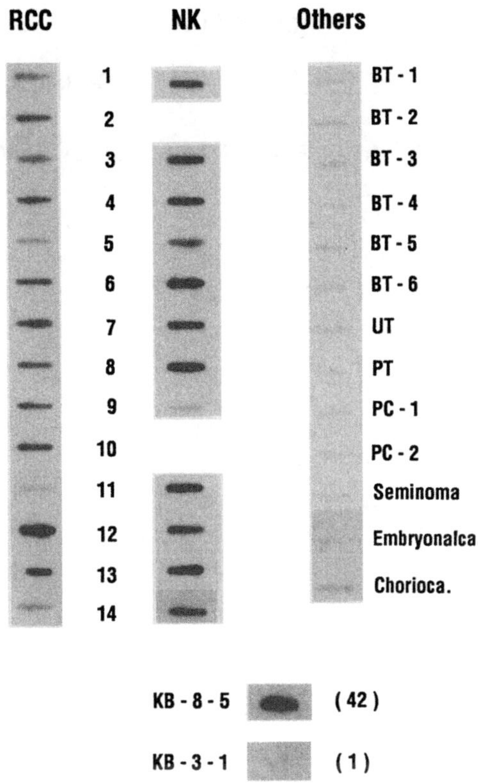

Fig. 1. Slot blots of 14 renal cell carcinoma (*RCC*), 12 adjacent normal kidney tissues (*NK*), and 11 other urogenital tumors (*BT*, bladder tumor; *UT*, ureteral tumor; *PT*, pelvic tumor; *PC*, prostatic cancer). Some 10 μg of total cellular RNA were applied to each slot and hybridized with human MDR 1 cDNA fragment 5A

Correlation of the MDR1 mRNA Levels with the Grades of Differentiation

Figure 2 shows RNA slot blot analyses of MDR1 in 38 RCC samples of primary lesions. The arbitrary units of the MDR1 RNA levels were determined by comparing the intensities of the autoradiogram with those of the multidrug-resistant KB-8-5 cells and its drug-sensitive parent, KB-3-1 cells. The mean MDR1 RNA level in the 30 well-differentiated RCCs (grades 1–2) was significantly higher than that in the eight poorly differentiated ones (grades 3–4), as shown in Fig. 3. These results are compatible with the premise that the increased expression of the MDR1 gene in RCC originates from the elevated expression in renal proximal tubule cells. There was no correlation, however, between MDR1 RNA levels and pathological T stage of the primary tumors. Figure 4 shows the comparison of MDR1 RNA levels in primary and metastatic lesions in four patients. The MDR1 RNA levels in the metastatic lesions were much higher than those in the primary lesions in two

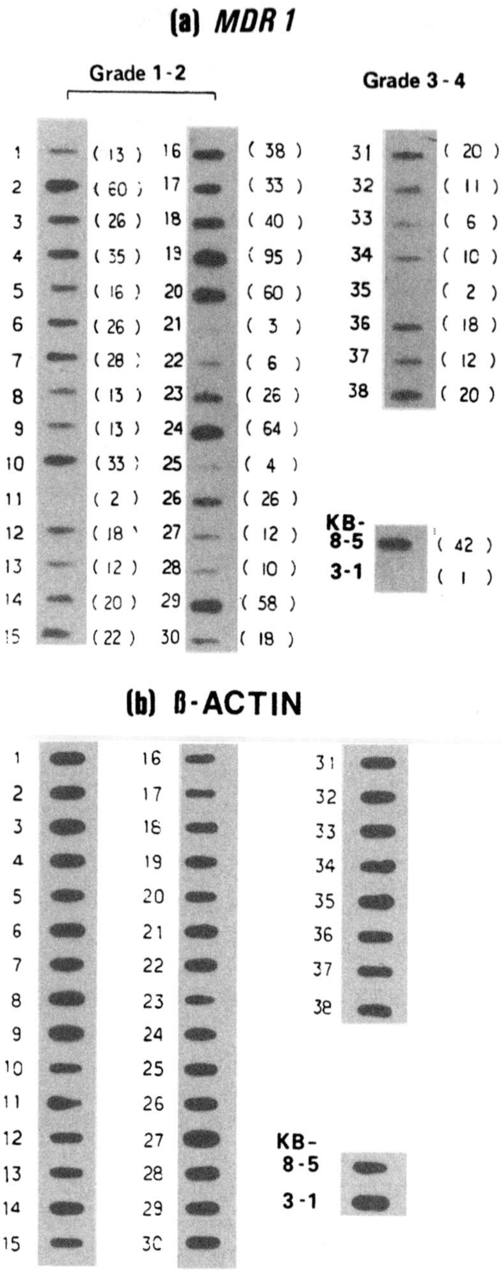

Fig. 2. a Slot blot analyses of RNA extracted from 38 samples of primary renal cell carcinoma lesions. Patients' numbers are shown on the *left side* of each slot. The arbitrary units of MDR1 RNA levels are shown in *parentheses*. **b** Slot blot analyses of RNA; same comparison, but filter was rehybridized with human β-actin pseudogene probe (pVB 2.1) after removal of the MDR1 probe

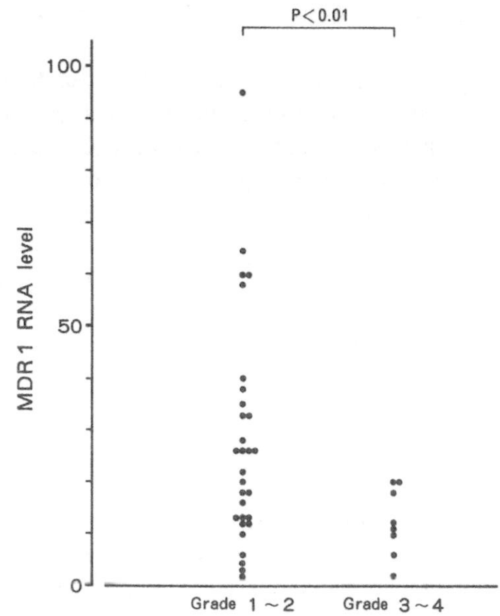

Fig. 3. Distribution of MDR1 RNA levels in 38 renal cell carcinomas by grade of lesion. Mean level for 30 well-differentiated ones (grades 1–2) was significantly higher than that for 8 poorly differentiated ones (grades 3–4) by the nonpaired Student's *t*-test

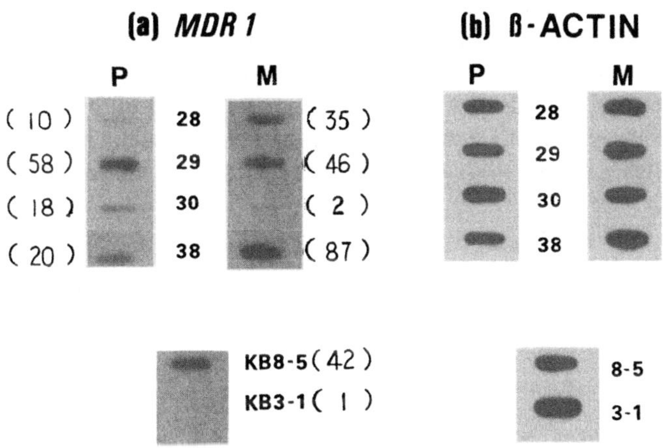

Fig. 4a,b. Slot blot analyses of RNA. **a** Comparison of MDR1 RNA levels in primary (*P*) and metastatic (*M*) lesions of patients 28, 29, 30, and 38. **b** Same comparison, but filter was rehybridized with β-actin probe

patients. Whether clones with higher MDR1 RNA levels are preferably selected in metastatic lesions remains to be elucidated.

In colchicine-selected KB cell lines, transcription of the MDR1 gene started from two promoter regions. In order to study which promoter was used in RCCs, we analyzed 12 RCC samples including metastatic lesions by the ribonuclease protection assay. The downstream promoter was mainly used in both primary and metastatic RCC samples [6].

Comparison Between MDR1 RNA Levels and In Vitro Chemosensitivity

To investigate the relationship between MDR1 RNA levels and drug sensitivity of tumors, we performed in vitro chemosensitivity testing using tumor explants of several types of cancers with various MDR1 RNA levels. The anticancer agents we tested were vinblastine, doxorubicin, and cisplatin. Sensitivity to each drug was defined as percentage inhibition of [^{3}H]-thymidine incorporation in a modified human tumor stem cell assay. These comparative studies, although preliminary, revealed that there was an inverse correlation between MDR1 RNA levels and in vitro vinblastine sensitivity, as shown in Fig. 5. There was no correlation of MDR1 RNA levels with either doxorubicin or cisplatin sensitivity.

Sensitizing Effect of Quinidine on De Novo Doxorubicin Resistance

Some calcium-channel blockers and calmodulin antagonists, quinidine, and several other agents are known to reverse the multidrug-resistance phenotype in vitro [8]. Fojo et al. reported that quinidine, at a clinically achievable concentration, remarkably enhanced sensitivity to vinblastine in several kidney cancer cell lines that are naturally multidrug-resistant [9]. We examined the enhancing effect of quinidine on sensitivity to doxorubicin in tumor explants from 16 RCC samples in relation to MDR1 gene expression [10]. We arbitrarily divided these samples into two groups, with the cutoff at an MDR1 RNA level of 20. Sensitivity to doxorubicin was significantly enhanced by the addition of quinidine (7.5 μg/ml) in RCCs with higher MDR1 RNA levels. On the contrary, the enhancing effect of quinidine was

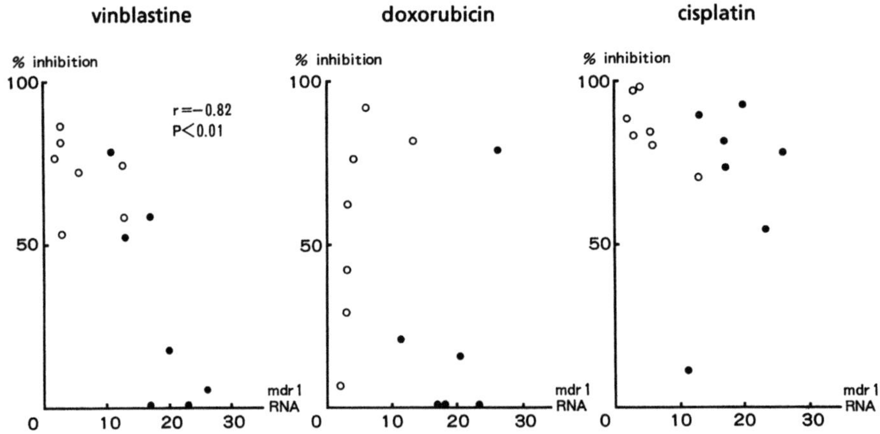

Fig. 5. Relationship between MDR1 RNA levels in each tumor and in vitro vinblastine, doxorubicin, and cisplatin sensitivities. In vitro drug sensitivity was assessed by percentage inhibition of (^{3}H)-thymidine incorporation. *Filled circles* are renal cell carcinomas, and *open circles* are other cancers

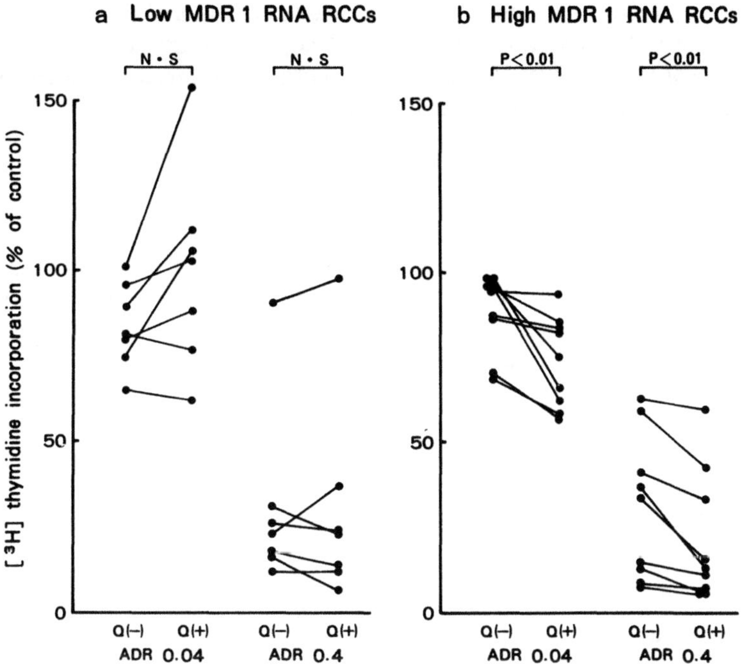

Fig. 6a,b. Effect of 7.5 μg/ml quinidine on in vitro sensitivity to doxorubicin (*ADR*) in 16 renal cell carcinoma (*RCC*) samples, which were divided into a group with low levels of MDR1 RNA (< 20) (**a**) or a group with high MDR1 RNA levels (> 20) (**b**). *N.S.*, not statistically significant; *Q*-, absence of quinidine; *Q*+, presence of quinidine

not statistically significant in RCCs with lower MDR1 RNA levels, as shown in Fig. 6. These results suggest that P170 contributes to not only vinblastine but also to doxorubicin de novo resistance in RCCs. At the same time, however, our data suggest that complex mechanisms [11, 12] other than P170 are also associated with doxorubicin resistance in RCCs.

Clinical Trials to Overcome Multidrug Resistance

Cardiac drugs such as verapamil in combination with *Vinca* alkaloids or anthracyclines have been preliminarily tried for patients with refractory leukemia and ovarian cancer. Favorable results were observed in children with acute lymphocytic leukemia [13], whereas a very poor response and severe cardiac toxicity were reported in patients with ovarian cancer [14]. Based on the results described above, we treated three patients with metastatic RCC with vinblastine or doxorubicin in combination with quinidine. No objective responses were observed, although almost the same serum concentration of quinidine as was applied in the in vitro studies could be achieved without any obvious cardiac or other complications. The

National Cancer Institute, USA, has started clinical trials using quinidine or amiodarone combined with doxorubicin and etoposide against RCC as well as colon and adrenal cancers. We think that such clinical trials aimed at overcoming multidrug resistance should be pursued as a high priority.

Conclusions

To summarize these data, the elevated expression of the MDR1 gene in RCC is possibly associated with de novo resistance to not only vinblastine but also doxorubicin. Our results, however, do not indicate that the combination of quinidine with doxorubicin is the best one for clinical use to overcome multidrug resistance in RCC, since the sensitizing effect of quinidine in RCC explants was not as remarkable as that observed in established cell lines. Mechanisms other than P170 can be also related to the multidrug-resistance phenomenon. Nevertheless, the present study does offer a possible approach to the development of new combination chemotherapy of clinical value in the treatment of RCC.

References

1. Chen C, Chin JE, Ueda K, Clark DP, Pastan I, Gottesman MM, Roninson I (1986) Internal duplication and homology with bacterial transport proteins in the MDR1 (P-glycoprotein) gene from multidrug-resistant human cells. Cell 47:381–349
2. Fojo AT, Akiyama S, Gottesman MM, Pastan I (1985) Reduced drug accumulation in multiply drug-resistant human KB carcinoma cell lines. Cancer Res 45:3002–3007
3. Fojo AT, Ueda K, Slamon DJ, Poplack DG, Gottesman MM, Pastan I (1987) Expression of a multidrug-resistance gene in human tumors and tissues. Proc Natl Acad Sci USA 84:265–269
4. Thiebaut F, Tsuruo T, Hamada H, Gottesman MM, Pastan I, Willinham MC (1987) Cellular localization of the multidrug-resistance gene product P-glycoprotein in normal human tissues. Proc Natl Acad Sci USA 84:7735–7738
5. Kakehi Y, Kanamaru H, Yoshida O, Ohkubo H, Nakanishi S, Gottesman MM, Pastan I (1988) Measurement of multidrug-resistance messenger RNA in urogenital cancers; elevated expression in renal cell carcinoma is associated with intrinsic drug resistance. J Urol 139:862–865
6. Ueda K, Yamano Y, Kioka N, Kakehi Y, Yoshida O, Gottesman MM, Pastan I, Komano T (1989) Detection of multidrug resistance (MDR1) gene expression in human tumors by a sensitive ribonuclease protection assay. Jpn J Cancer Res 80:1127–1132
7. Friedman HM, Glaubiger DL (1982) Assessment of in vitro drug sensitivity of human tumor cells using [^{3}H]thymidine incorporation in a modified human tumor stem cell assay. Cancer Res 42:4683–4689
8. Tsuruo T, Iida H, Tsukagoshi S, Sakurai Y (1982) Increased accumulation of vincristine and adriamycin in drug-resistant P388 tumor cells following incubation with calcium antagonists and calmodulin inhibitors. Cancer Res 42:4730–4733
9. Fojo AT, Shen D-W, Mickley LA, Pastan I, Gottesman MM (1987) Intrinsic drug resistance in human kidney cancer is associated with expression of a human multidrug-resistance gene. J Clin Oncol 5:1922–1927

10. Kanamaru H, Kakehi Y, Yoshida O, Nakanishi S, Pastan I, Gottesman MM (1989) MDR1 RNA levels in human renal cell carcinomas: correlation with grade and prediction of reversal of doxorubicin resistance by quinidine in tumor explants. J Natl Cancer Inst 81:844–849
11. Kramer RA, Zakher J, Kim G (1988) Role of the glutathione redox cycle in acquired and de novo multidrug resistance. Science 241:694–697
12. Tsuruo T (1988) Mechanisms of multidrug resistance and implications for therapy. Jpn J Cancer Res 79:285–296
13. Bessho F, Kinumaki H, Kobayashi M, Habu H, Yokota S, Tsuruo T, Kobayashi N (1985) Treatment of children with refractory acute lymphocytic leukemia with vincristine and diltiazem. Med Pediat Oncol 13:199–202
14. Ozols RF, Cunnion RE, Klecker RW Jr, Hamilton TC, Osatchega Y, Parrilo JE, Young RC (1987) Verapamil and adriamycin in the treatment of drug-resistant ovarian cancer patients. J Clin Oncol 5:641–647

Radioimmunoconjugates in Renal Cell Carcinoma

R.L. Vessella[1]

Introduction

The long-awaited clinical benefits of radioimmunoscintigraphy (RIS) and radioimmunotherapy (RIT) are being realized in a slow but steadily progressive fashion [1]. The visualization of tumor foci no longer requires extensive manipulative steps to discriminate uptake of radiolabeled antibody by the tumor from that of the blood pool or normal tissues, and in therapeutic regimens significant tumor responses are becoming more common. However, the past decade of animal studies and clinical efforts utilizing radionuclide conjugated monoclonal antibodies (MAb) has demonstrated the vast complexities of the task at hand, and even as enthusiasm is growing, significant hurdles remain to be cleared if RIS and RIT are to achieve their anticipated clinical potential. We have been actively exploring the use of RIS and RIT in renal cell carcinoma (RCC) xenografts for 5 years and in clinical trials for approximately 2 years. This report will briefly review the progress to date and then in more detail will provide an overview of the key RIS and RIT issues that are being addressed by the scientific community.

RCC was selected nearly 10 years ago as the target for RIS and RIT studies for several reasons:

a) There existed no established treatment for metastatic disease so that even a modest response rate from RIT would be beneficial;
b) staging could be improved if RIS proved successful in detecting occult masses refractory to current imaging modalities;
c) efforts to produce MAbs suitable for RIS and RIT might also lead to MAbs which would detect a RCC serum/urine tumor associated marker;
d) RCC appears to respond more to immunological intervention than most other solid tumors, and one could argue that the necrotic areas in the tumor as well as the documented spontaneous remissions have an immunological basis; and
e) thanks to prior efforts by former colleagues at the University of Minnesota where this work was performed, several RCC cell lines and RCC xenografts were readily available for use in these studies [2, 3].

[1] University of Washington Medical Center, Department of Urology RL-10, Seattle, WA 98195, USA

F.M.J. Debruyne et al. (Eds.)
Immunotherapy of Renal Cell Carcinoma

Results

From the dozens of MAbs generated to RCC, four (designated A6H, B4F, C5H, and D5D) were selected for extensive in vivo studies involving RCC xenografts (designated TK-39, TK-82, TK-177, and TK-201) implanted subcutaneously or under the renal capsule in athymic mice [4–6]. MAbs A6H, C5H, and D5D were of the IgG1 subclass and B4F was available as IgG2a and IgG2b subclasses. The detailed methodologies used in the xenograft studies have been published elsewhere [7]. In general, subcutaneous xenografts ranged in size from 40–240 mg and those implanted under the renal capsule from approximately 5 to 50 mg. MAbs were purified using protein A affinity chromatography from sodium sulfate cuts of ascitic fluids and radiolabeled with iodine 131 or iodine 125 using the chloramine T procedure to a specific activity of approximately 5 μCi/μg. The immunological reactivity of the radiolabeled MAb was verified prior to injection using a live cell binding assay. For our clinical studies, a phase I-II Investigational New Drug application (IND) was prepared in accordance with Food and Drug Administration (FDA) guidelines. MAb A6H was produced in collaboration with Abbott Laboratories (Chicago, IL) in an air lift fermenter and purified by protein A chromatography. The purified material was checked for viral, endotoxin, and protein A contaminants prior to radiolabeling at the VA Medical Center in Minneapolis. Following iodination, the antibody was checked for immunological reactivity as indicated and assayed for the presence of aggregates by high-pressure liquid chromatography (HPLC). Endotoxin tests were performed again prior to infusion.

Our experience with RCC RIS in the xenograft model has been remarkably successful as documented by the ability to detect tumor sites as small as 7 mg with MAb A6H, which has performed somewhat better than the other three MAbs in vivo. Likewise, our initial RIT studies were successful and among the first to document long-term regression of solid tumor xenografts using patient equivalent activity doses of [^{131}I]-labeled MAbs. A summary of these early RIS and RIT efforts has been published [8].

During the past 2 years we have investigated several aspects of RIT, including a comparison of tumor responses from RIT to that achieved with acute dose external beam radiation therapy (XRT) [9]. RIT differs from XRT through the delivery of irradiation at an ultra low dose rate (< 0.5 cGy/min) over a continuous period of several days. The consequences of this low dose rate on tumor response are not well known, but this aspect of RIT and other related issues have been the topic of several recent reviews [10–12].

Our experiences to date can be summarized as follows: There exists a stratified radiobiological response among the xenografts (TK-39<TK-82<TK-177), which is observed with RIT and XRT. The MAb deposition patterns would appear to correlate well with the achieved radiobiological responses, ranging from the most heterogeneous in TK-39 to nearly homogeneous in TK-177. Recent results show a difference in the vascular permeability of the RCC xenografts and an interesting correlation with the stratified radiobiological responses. In another study, encouraging results were obtained from combining XRT with RIT; tumor control was

achieved in TK-39, which was not possible with any single modality [13]. Many of these studies illustrate well the complexity of RIT and the significant influence of the microenvironment. Nevertheless, the results favorably suggest that heretofore radioresistant solid tumors may respond to combined radiotherapy approaches. The radiobiological mechanisms that govern the tumor response to ultra low dose rate irradiation are unknown but will be the subject of future investigations and discussions.

Based on successes in the RCC xenograft model, an IND was acquired for a phase I-II RIS and RIT clinical trial of MAb A6H in patients with RCC. This work was performed in collaboration with Abbott Laboratories. Initially, the RIS protocol involved the administration of [^{131}I]-labeled whole molecule A6H at an activity dose of 5 mCi (mass dose of 5, 10, 20, or 40 mg MAb). If tumor foci were successfully imaged as defined in the IND, then we proceeded with RIT at an administered dose of 50 mCi and equivalent mass dose. The first several patients showed unexpectedly fast clearance of the labeled MAb ($T_{1/2}$ of less than 10 h) and poor uptake by the tumor site(s), although five patients had positive tumor images [14]. For example, in Fig. 1, an infusion of 20 mg [^{131}I]-labeled A6H resulted in the visualization of two sites in this 66-year-old man: the primary RCC in the left kidney and a metastatic abdominal mass. Based on a review of the data and preliminary investigations, two posibilities were put forward as explanations for the fast serum clearance:

a) the antigen or some interfering substance in the serum was promoting rapid uptake by the reticuloendothelial system, or
b) MAb A6H was reacting strongly with accessible normal tissue antigens.

The former problem was easier to solve and was addressed first. Two approaches were taken: A6H was infused as F(ab')2 fragments to minimize uptake by the reticuloendothelial system via the Fc portion of the antibody, and then this was preceded by a preinfusion of unlabeled A6H as a "scavenger" for interfering substances in the serum. The preinfusion approach followed by F(ab')2 fragments succeeded in

Table 1. Phase I-II radioimmunoscintigraphy with A6H escalation and "scavenger" series

Dose infused (mg)	(+) Image	(–) Image
Intact antibody:		
5	0	3
10	2	2
20	3	2
40	0	3
F(ab')2:		
5	0	2
Scavenger:		
10 intact + 10 intact	2	6
10 intact + 10 F(ab')2	6	2

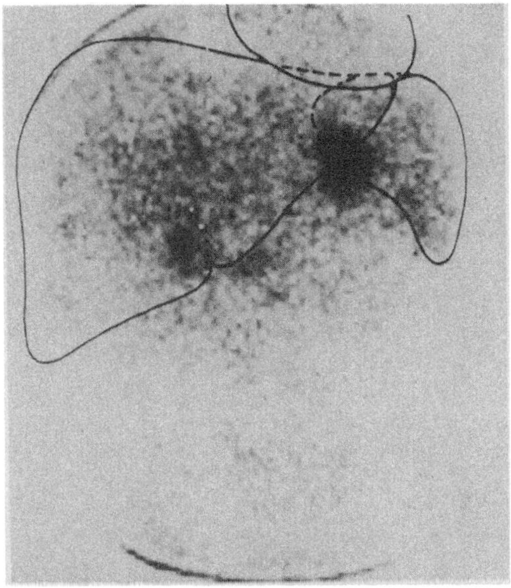

Fig. 1. A 66-year-old man presented with primary (left kidney) and metastatic (abdominal) renal cell carcinoma. This patient had received no prior treatment. He was given a 20 mg infusion of [^{131}I]-labeled MAb A6H (19 mg unlabeled plus 1 mg labeled; 5 mCi). Planar images were acquired at days 1 and 4 post infusion, with the 4-day image displayed here. Primary and metastatic disease sites were visualized

prolonging the serum clearance rates and significantly improved the targeting of tumor sites [15]. Figure 2 is a planar image of a woman with metastatic RCC in the hip. This particular site was also detected by computerized axial tomography (CAT), and at a subsequent RIT infusion of 50 mCi, SPECT analysis confirmed the planar scans. Summarizing these clinical RIS efforts, 33 evaluable studies were performed using either the dose escalation approach with whole MAb, F(ab')2 MAb, or the scavenger series (Table 1). The best results were observed with the scavenger protocol using a mass dose of 10 mg of radiolabeled F(ab')2 A6H. Six of eight patients in this investigative arm of the protocol were scored as image positive.

RIT was performed in four patients at the lowest therapy dose of 50 mCi [^{131}I]-labeled F(ab')2 A6H using the scavenger approach. Dosimetry estimates were performed on three of the four patients. As shown in Table 2, 1300, 1040, and 55 cGy were delivered to the three evaluable tumor sites. In all of the RIT study patients, the estimated absorbed dose to the bone marrow was < 25 cGy. The patient with the highest estimated tumor absorbed dose had an inoperable recurrent mass in the left splenic bed following a prior nephrectomy and splenectomy plus extensive periaortic adenopathy. Uptake of the radioimmunoconjugate by the periaortic mass was not evaluable because of interference from residual liver uptake. During the weeks following RIT, the splenic bed mass regressed, and residual disease became

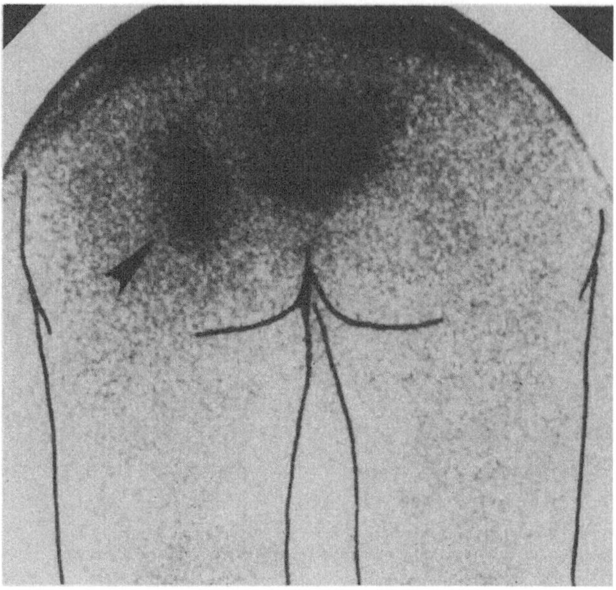

Fig. 2. A 55-year-old woman presented with metastatic renal cell carcinoma in the left hilum and bone. Patient received a 10 mg, unlabeled, A6H infusion immediately followed by a 10 mg [^{131}I]-labeled F(ab')2 A6H (9 mg unlabeled A6H plus 1 mg labeled A6H; 5 mCi) infusion. Planar images were acquired on days 1 and 4 post infusion, with the 4-day image of hip joint metastasis shown here. An image of the bladder from catabolised [^{131}I]-labeled A6H is also noted. This particular bone metastasis was confirmed by CAT scans and at a subsequent RIT dose of [^{131}I]-labeled A6H (50 mCi), the site was clearly seen by SPECT

Table 2. A synopsis of the radioimmunotherapy clinical trials using a 50 mCi infusion (antibody mass doses provided in the table). The tumor-absorbed irradiation dose in the three evaluable patients is presented. The 175 g mass in patient 240A regressed following RIT and was undetectable for 24 months. The remaining three patients progressed rapidly and have died

Patient	Tumor location	Tumor mass (g estimated)	% injected dose (42 h)	% injected dose (67 h)	Dose* (rads)
240A	Splenic bed	175	7	10	1300
509T	Upper lift hilum	63.5	7	8	1040
563C	Upper pole right kidney	65		4	
576P	Skull	33.5	0.15	0.25	53

* Dose to bone marrow in all patients < 25 rads

undetectable. The other mass remained unremarkable and was removed surgically. Exploration of the left splenic bed at the time of surgery failed to detect the presence of residual RCC. It is noteworthy that the tumor removed during surgery was mostly A6H antigen-negative on immunohistochemical analysis (see subsequent discussion on issue of antigen heterogeneity). The patient was followed up regularly, and for 24 months there was no evidence of disease – an abdominal recurrence has now been noted.

Although one would not expect RCC to respond to 1300 cGy, the heterogeneous nature of radiolabeled MAb deposition in solid tumors may in fact impart manyfold higher absorbed doses to subpopulations of tumor cells, particularly those surrounding the neovasculature. Also, extrapolating from recent xenograft studies, the response to low dose rate irradiation may be greater than previously believed. The patient (509T) whose tumor site received ~1000 cGy showed no significant response and soon expired from massive metastatic disease. All of the patients tolerated the 50 mCi dose without signs of bone marrow depression or other significant side effects. Accordingly, with tumor:bone marrow ratios > 40:1 in two of the three evaluable patients, there appears justification to increase the infused dose incrementally to a level at which dosimetry estimates to the marrow stabilize between 150 and 200 cGy.

Issues of Importance

The advances being made in RIS and RIT are due to the interdisciplinary efforts of many investigators. Early difficulties with RIS or RIT were attributed to insufficient immunological specificity, and indeed, exhaustive efforts in this area have contributed to better results. However, it also became apparent that no single discipline possessed the necessary expertise to unravel the complex behavior of these labeled products in vivo. At least eleven issues have been identified as being critically relevant to the successful clinical implementation of RIS and/or RIT, including

a) choice of radionuclide,
b) route of injection,
c) pharmacokinetics,
d) accessibility of the solid tumors to the antibody as a function of vascularity and vascular permeability,
e) distribution of the antibody within the tumor,
f) antigen distribution, modulation, and secretion,
g) mode of detecting antibody targeting,
h) dosimetry at a cellular level,
i) radiobiology of ultra low dose rate irradiation,
j) normal tissue toxicities, and
k) control or avoidance of the human antimouse response.

Some of these issues will be addressed in more detail.

Identification of the "best" radionuclide(s) for conjugation with the tumor-reactive MAb for RIS and RIT remains an active area of debate [16]. Numerous choices exist, some are suitable for imaging (e.g., ^{99}Tc, ^{131}I, ^{111}In) or therapy (^{131}I, ^{90}Y, ^{186}Re) and a select few such as ^{131}I and possibly ^{186}Re are useful in both applications. In general, of the methodologies used to radiolabel an antibody for in vivo application, radioiodination is the most common due to the relatively gentle nature of the technique, ready commercial availability of the isotope, and well-understood catabolic mechanisms. The gamma energy spectrums of ^{99}Tc and ^{111}In are better suited for RIS, but stable antibody conjugation requires sophisticated techniques, many of which are proprietary. Similar problems confront the use of beta-emitting radionuclides other than ^{131}I for therapy.

A disappointment in the clinical trials to date has been the lower than anticipated accumulation of radiolabeled MAb at the tumor site when compared with results previously obtained in the preclinical model. In fact, the concentration of MAb at the tumor site (0.1%–0.001% injected dose/g) may be several log magnitudes below that seen in xenografts. Many factors contribute to these findings, of which the dilution of antibody upon intravenous administration is a major consideration. Accordingly, alternative routes of administration have been used in certain situations to deliver selectively a higher concentration of the antibody to the tumor site. For example, improved targeting of ovarian tumors has been achieved by switching from an intravenous route to intraperitoneal administration [17]. In tumors having a direct venous input, infusion of the MAb via the supplying arterial vessel has been considered.

A discussion of the multiple pharmacokinetic and microenvironmental factors that affect the performance of MAbs in vivo is beyond the scope of this report, but the interested reader is referred to two excellent reviews of the subject [18, 19]. Generally, any factor that influences the clearance of antibody from the circulation, the targeting of the tumor, the distribution within the tumor, and the rate/method of catabolism, including the fate of the radionuclide following catabolism, can significantly affect the ultimate therapeutic potential of radioimmunoconjugates. Studies of biodistribution are critical in determining the MAb pharmacokinetics. However, whereas such studies are easily performed in the animal model, detection of antibody distribution in humans is much more difficult and must rely on relatively insensitive imaging techniques and tissue biopsies. The serum clearance rates of MAb conjugates have ranged from hours to several days, and any given MAb may or may not show prolonged clearance rates as the mass dose is increased. Any subtle change in the antibody, such as the method of radiolabeling, can dramatically alter the biodistribution. Alternatively, manipulation of the antibody's pharmacokinetics may provide very powerful mechanisms of improving image resolution and tumoricidal effects.

Logic dictates that if the infused antibody reacted with a circulating tumor-associated antigen, little if any of the antibody would reach the tumor site – the antibody/antigen complexes would be efficiently eliminated from the circulation by the reticuloendothelial system. However, in numerous studies involving the tumor antigen CEA, there has been little interference seen from circulating antigen. Also, the targeting of membrane antigens is no guarantee of success, especially if the targeted antigen is expressed at low concentrations ($< 10^6$ copies per cell) if it modulates (primarily a concern for lymphoid antigens), or if the expression is heterogeneous among cells of the tumor population. The latter occurs frequently within solid tumors and is one reason why radionuclides conjugated to MAbs, with a broad cellular range of cytotoxicity, may be preferential to drug-immunoconjugates. One of the more complex issues involved in RIT is predicting and quantitating the absorbed tumor radiation dose. Dosimetric calculations incorporate the energy of the radionuclide, duration of exposure, and amount of radionuclide deposited at the tissue site. Following RIT, assessments of exposure and amount of radionuclide at the tumor site are not easy to acquire due to the pharmacokinetics of tumor targeting and the assumed heterogeneous deposition of MAb within the tumor. In addition, there is uncertainty in the calculation of the absorbed dose to the bone marrow from RIT, the organ system most at risk from radiation toxicity.

One concern which may be the most limiting to the eventual use of RIT as a continual therapeutic modality in humans is the generation of human antimouse antibodies (HAMA) following the initial infusion of MAbs. Reports vary as to the limitations which HAMA has imposed on current clinical trials, although most have not involved very many infusions. Alternate approaches, such as derivation of tumor-reactive human MAbs have been relatively unsuccessful. However, limited trials with chimeric MAbs which are part mouse (antigen binding portion of the molecule) and part human (Fc portion) have shown signs of promise. Advances in the field of genetic engineering will continue to contribute to these endeavors.

In conclusion, many of the factors impacting on the eventual implementation of RIS and RIT have been identified and are being addressed in multidiscipline efforts by numerous research teams. RCC appears as an especially attractive target for MAb immunoconjugate interventions. We believe that combined therapeutic modalities will be more successful than RIT by itself and that the heretofore radioresistant nature of RCC should not preclude active XRT/RIT efforts. Moreover, RIT and chemotherapeutic drug (e.g., 5 fluorouracil) combinations may prove efficacious if current studies in this laboratory show an effect of ultra low dose rate irradiation on cell cycle synchrony.

Acknowledgements. This work could not have been attempted without the enormous support of my colleagues, collaborators, postdoctoral fellows, graduate students, and technical staff. Space does not allow an individualized listing of these critical personnel, but special recognition is given to Paul Lange, M.D., Mike Elson, Ph.D., Rei Chiou, M.D., Frank Grund, M.D., Debra Lightner, M.D., Barry Wessels, Ph.D, Timothy Johnson, Ph.D., and Donald Palme. In addition, funding for these projects was provided by the Veterans Administration the Minnesota Medical Foundation, and Abbott Laboratories. This support is greatly appreciated.

References

1. Larson SM (1990) Clinical radioimmunodetection, overview and suggestions for standardization of clinical trials. Cancer Res 50 (Suppl):892–898
2. Clayman RV, Figenshau RS, Bear A, Limas C (1985) Transplantation of human renal cell carcinoma into athymic mice. Cancer Res 45:2650–2653
3. Williams RD, Elliot AY, Stein N, et al. (1978) In vitro cultivation of human renal cell cancer. In Vitro 14:779–786
4. Vessella R, Moon T, Chiou R, Nowak J, Arfman E, Palme D, Peterson G, Lange p (1985) Monoclonal antibodies to human renal cell carcinoma: Recognition of shared and restricted antigens. Cancer Res 45:6131–6139
5. Chiou RK, Vessella RL, Elson MK, Clayman RV, Gonzalez-Campoy J, Klicka MJ, Shafer RB, Lange PH (1985) Localization of human renal cell carcinoma xenografts with a tumor-preferential monoclonal antibody. Cancer Res 45:6140–6146
6. Moon T, Vessella R, Palme D, Nowak J, Lange P (1985) A highly restricted antigen for renal cell carcinoma defined by a monoclonal antibody. Hybridoma 4:163–171
7. Vessella RL, Lange PH, Palme DF, Chiou RK, Elson MK, Wessels BW (1988) Radioiodinated monoclonal antibodies in the imaging and treatment of human renal cell carcinoma xenografts in nude mice. In: Rodwell JD (ed) Antibody-mediated delivery systems. Dekker, New York, pp 245–282
8. Vessella R, Alvarez V, Chiou R, Rodwell J, Elson M, Palme D, Shafer R, Lange P (1987) Radioimmunoscintigraphy and radioimmunotherapy of renal cell carcinoma xenografts. NCI Monographs 3:159–167
9. Wessels VW, Vessella RL, Palme DF, Berkopec JM, Smith GK, Bradley EW (1989) Radiobiological comparison of external beam irradiation and radioimmunotherapy in renal cell carcinoma xenografts. Int J Radiotion Oncology Biol Phys 17:1257–1263
10. Wessels BW (1990) Current status of animal radioimmunotherapy. Cancer Res 50 (Suppl): 970s–973s
11. Langmuir VK, Sutherland RM (1988) Radiobiology of radioimmunotherapy: Current status. Antibody Immunocon Radiophar 1(3):195–211
12. Humm JL, Cobb LM (1990) Nonuniformity of tumor dose in radioimmunotherapy. J Nucl Med 31:75–83
13. Berkopec JM, Bradley BW, Wessels DF, Palme DF, Montilla L, Vessella RL (1989) Combined external beam irradiation (XRT) and radioimmunotherapy (RIT) on renal cell carcinoma xenografts. J Nucl Med 30 (5):406
14. Vessella RL, Chiou RK, Grund FM, Elson MK, Johnson TK, Nowak JA, Palme DF, Lightner DJ, Mathisen ML, Wessels BW, Olson RE, Rittenhouse HG, Stroup SD, Lange PH (1987) Renal cell carcinoma (RCC) phase I-II trials with 131-I labeled monoclonal antibody A6H: Imaging and pharmacokinetic studies. Proc Am Assoc Cancer Res 28:1525
15. Lightner DJ, Vessella RL, Chiour RK, Grund FM, Johnson TK, Elson MK, Wessels BW, Stroupe SD, Mathisen ML, Lange PH (1988) Renal cell carcinoma phase I-II trials with I-131 monoclonal antibody (MoAb) A6H. Proc Third International Conference on Monoclonal Antibody Immunoconjugates for Cancer, vol 92, p 119
16. Wessels VW, Rogus RP (1984) Radionuclide selection and model absorbed dose calculations for radiolabeled tumor associated antibodies. Med Phys 11:638–645
17. Griffin TW, Collins J, Bokhari F, Stochl M, Brill AB, Ito T, Emond G, Sands H (1990) Intraperitoneal immunoconjugates. Cancer Res 50 (Suppl):1031s–1038s
18. Sands H (1990) Experimental studies of radioimmunodetection of cancer: An overview. Cancer Res 50 (Suppl):809s–813s
19. Jain RK (1990) Physiological barriers to delivery of monoclonal antibodies and other macromolecules in tumors. Cancer Res 50 (Suppl):814s–819s

Interferon and Tumor Necrosis Factor in Renal Cell Carcinoma Model Systems

R.J.A. van Moorselaar, A.J.M.C. Beniers, J.A. Schalken, and F.M.J. Debruyne[1]

Introduction

Renal cell carcinoma (RCC) is the most common kidney tumor in adults. The incidence peak is found in the sixth decade of life [34]. Approximately 25%–30% of patients with RCC have metastases at the time of diagnosis [10]. Furthermore, metastases develop in a majority of untreated patients within 1 year after discovery. Advanced RCC is refractory to nearly all forms of systemic therapy. Hormonal therapy may result in a small proportion (0%–10%) of objective responses, but these are incomplete and of short duration. Single or combination chemotherapy also yields no clearly definable improvement in patient survival [19].

Immunotherapy is a relatively new approach in cancer therapy. Interest in immunologic approaches has been fostered by the rare but well-documented observations of spontaneous regression of metastases after nephrectomy [16]. These observations suggest that host factors may be capable of modifying the course of RCC.

Immunotherapy is divided into two overlapping categories, active and passive [11, 14]. In direct or specific active immunotherapy the host antitumor immunity, either cellular or humoral, is stimulated against a certain tumor by using tumor vaccines. In RCC, active immunotherapy using irradiated tumor cells with candida antigen as adjuvant, could not statistically alter the prognosis compared to an age-matched control group [30]. Active nonspecific immunotherapy has been used to activate immune response mechanisms in a generalized manner. Substances used in this regard have included BCG, interferon and other lymphokines. Passive immunotherapy includes antitumor antisera, monoclonal antibodies directed specifically against tumor antigens and adoptive cellular immunotherapy. In the last-mentioned treatment the patient's peripheral blood lymphocytes or lymphocytes extracted from tumors are exposed to interleukin-2 (IL-2) in vitro to proliferate to lymphokine-activated killer cells (LAK cells) [13, 32] or tumor-infiltrating lymphocytes (TIL cells) [4] and then transferred back into the host together with additional IL-2.

Today, the interferons (IFN) are the most extensively studied biological response modifiers (BRM) in metastatic RCC. The IFNs are a group of naturally occurring

[1] Department of Urology, University Hospital Nijmegen, P.O. Box 9101, 6500 HB Nijmegen, The Netherlands

F.M.J. Debruyne et al. (Eds.)
Immunotherapy of Renal Cell Carcinoma

proteins with potent antiviral, antiproliferative and immunomodulatory properties such as activation of natural killer cells and macrophages and modulation of class I and II HLA antigens [35]. On the basis of their antigenic properties a division is made into three main groups. The α-IFNs are a group of closely related proteins with approximately 75% homology in their amino acid sequences. They are produced by macrophages and leukocytes upon exposure to virus particles and compete with β-IFN for the same receptor. γ-IFN is the product of a single gene and is produced by activated T-lymphocytes.

Tumor necrosis factor alpha (TNF), originally identified as a substance produced by macrophages exposed to endotoxin [8], possesses a number of biological activities, particularly antitumor activity. TNF causes cytostasis or cytolysis of in vitro cell cultures from a variety of animal and human malignant tumors [36] and tumor necrosis in tumor-bearing animals [8].

As shown for other solid tumors, different combinations of α- and γ-IFN and TNF can result in the enhancement of their respective antitumor activities in vitro [9, 15, 22] and in vivo [3, 33, 37]. We have performed in vitro studies using five RCC xenografts [5] and in vivo studies with eight RCC xenografts [6] and a rat renal cell tumor model system [39] to assess the direct and indirect antiproliferative effects of BRMs in RCC. In this manuscript we will describe in brief the different experiments and their respective results.

Experimental Studies in RCC: Our Own Observations

To investigate the antiproliferative effects of α- and γ-IFN and TNF we have used in vitro and in vivo model systems.

In Vitro Tests

In order to obtain insight into the direct inhibitory effects of the BRM on the proliferative capacity of renal tumor cells, in vitro tests were performed using five different RCC xenografts. After original subcutaneous transplantation of small pieces of tumor ($2\,mm^3$) in both flanks of Balb-C nu/nu mice, the tumors were passaged every 4 weeks. Single cell suspensions were used for in vitro tests using a soft agar colony-forming assay. Drugs were given as a single administration on day 1, and colony formation was followed for a period of 4 weeks during which growth was measured using temporal growth curves [12]. Dose-dependent inhibition in colony formation was evident for all five tumor lines in the single-drug tests. In combination tests, 1500 IU IFN/ml and 3000 IU TNF/ml were used. The results are summarized in Table 1. All combinations showed synergistic effects except for the combination of α-IFN and γ-IFN in the NC-65 tumor, which had subadditive effects. The combinations of IFN and TNF showed the best in vitro antiproliferative effects. Heterogeneity towards the direct antiproliferative effects of BRMs in RCC was shown. It is clear that from these data only limited conclusions

Table 1. Percentage survival of different xenografts after growth in soft agar and application of a single dose of BRM compared to the untreated control

Drug combination	Tumor RC-43	NC-65	NU-12	HAM-II	HAM-III
α-IFN	25	70	55	85	35
γ-IFN	45	90	30	90	95
TNF	55	75	40	35	25
α-IFN/γ-IFN	3	65	10	70	20
α-IFN/TNF	0	0	3	3	0
γ-IFN/TNF	20	2	4	3	8

IFN concentration, 1500 IU/ml; *TNF* concentration, 3000 IU/ml

can be drawn for the actual clinical setting because of the major effects on the immune system of the host; therefore it is necessary to do in vivo tests.

In Vivo Tests

For in vivo studies nude mice and rats were used. Heterotransplantation of human RCC onto nude mice is a suitable model to test the direct antiproliferative effects of BRMs; however, due to the lack of an intact immune system, the indirect, T-cell mediated, antitumor effects cannot be evaluated. To evaluate the contributions of the immune system a syngeneic rat renal cell carcinoma model system was used.

Eight human renal tumor xenografts were transplanted subcutaneously into nude mice [6]. Of three tested routes of administration, intravenous, intraperitoneal and subcutaneous only the subcutaneous route was effective against tumor growth. IFN was given 3 times per week and TNF 3 or 5 times per week in different concentrations. From initial results with the NC-65 tumor 10 treatment regimens were chosen, α-IFN 0.5 and 5 ng/gram mouse, γ-IFN 8 and 80 ng/gram and TNF 500 ng/gram were used and combinations of these BRMs in order to evaluate the effects in the other xenografts. Combinations of both α- and γ-IFN with TNF resulted in a complete growth inhibition of most tumors. All tested RCC xenografts showed different sensitivities towards the BRMs, which may represent the heterogeneity of RCC. The IFNs showed to have optimum doses, which was sometimes a low dose, TNF antitumor effects were dose-dependent. The best antiproliferative effects were found when treatment was started 24 h after tumor implantation, treatment starting at a tumor volume of 50 mm^3 showed no or slight growth inhibiting effects.

Human leukocyte antigen (HLA) molecules, encoded by the major histocompatibility complex (MHC), play a central regulatory role in the immune response. Preliminary studies showed that HLA class I was expressed by all untreated lines, while only two of eight lines expressed class II. The class I and class II expression can be augmented or induced, respectively, by BRM therapy. Investigations on

HLA expression patterns in BRM-sensitive and -insensitive tumors might give us insight into the mode of action of IFN and TNF.

In a rat renal cell carcinoma model system [23, 39] the antiproliferative activities of recombinant rat γ-IFN and recombinant human TNF were investigated. Rat γ-IFN had to be used because of the species specificity of IFN. The tumor was transplanted subcutaneously, the drugs were administered peritumorally. γ-IFN treatment starting 2 days after tumor implantation resulted in a dose-dependent growth-inhibiting effect. TNF was effective only at the highest concentration. Different combinations of the drugs had additive or synergistic antiproliferative effects (Table 2). The combination of both highest doses completely inhibited tumor growth. The antitumor effect was dependent on tumor volume at start of therapy. Monotherapy could not inhibit growth of an established tumor. The combination of both highest doses, however, stabilized tumor volume even when treatment was started at a tumor volume of 2–5 cm^3.

Synergistic antiproliferative effects of chemotherapeutic agents in combination with immunotherapy, e.g., etoposide (VP-16) and TNF [7] have been observed in nude mice. We have investigated another DNA topoisomerase II inhibitor, Adriamycin (Adria), in combination with TNF in vitro and in vivo [40]. In vitro studies were performed with a cell line established from the original rat renal cell tumor. Cells were plated at a concentration of 50 000 per dish in the upper layer of the double-layer soft-agar culture system. TNF and Adria were layered over the top agar in a volume of 200 μl. TNF (1 ng–1000 ng/dish) and Adria (2 ng–20 000 ng/dish) showed dose-dependent antiproliferative effects in vitro; different combinations had synergistic antiproliferative effects. For in vivo studies the rat tumor was transplanted subcutaneously and Adria was administered intraperitoneally, 0.1 or 1 mg/kg bodyweight, in different treatment schedules. The highest dose of Adria monotherapy, 1 mg/kg per day for 3 consecutive days every 2 weeks, showed significant antitumor effects. Other Adria regimens did not produce significant antitumor effects. Only in the combinations with the highest Adria dose were there synergistic antiproliferative effect with TNF. However, combination treatment was always significantly more effective than the respective monotherapies. Also, in these chemo-immunotherapy regimens it was shown that treatment starting at higher tumor loads had no significant antitumor effects.

Discussion and Prospects

Chemotherapy and radiotherapy have limited therapeutic efficacy in advanced RCC; therefore, new treatment modalities must be developed. In vitro studies have shown that BRMs such as α-IFN, γ-IFN and TNF have antiproliferative effects against RCC [5, 24]. The inhibitory effects of the BRMs varies with the RCC cell line, the differential sensitivity reflecting the heterogeneity of human RCC. In vivo studies in nude mice revealed a dose-dependent relationship for TNF and a bell-shaped response curve for IFN. In a review of α-IFN monotherapy the same was found for humans [26]. While in low-dose regimens fewer than 2% of evaluable patients dis-

Table 2. Effect of different doses of IFN or TNF, three and five times weekly respectively, and their combinations against a subcutaneous rat renal cell tumor

Therapy IFN (U)	TNF (μg)	Effect of combination	Inhibition on day 42 (%)[a]	Remission[b]
0	0	–	0	0/6
8 000	0	–	57	0/6
80 000	0	–	87	0/6
0	1	–	44	0/6
0	10	–	36	0/6
0	100	–	74	0/6
8 000	10	Additive	77	0/6
8 000	100	Additive	82	0/6
80 000	10	Synergistic	99	4/6
80 000	100	Synergistic	100	6/6

Start of treatment 48 h after tumor implantation
[a] Growth inhibition compared to untreated controls
[b] Cured rats/total rats per group

played responses and high-dose regimens yielded response rates of approximately 10%, the moderately toxic intermediate doses induced responses in 19% of 242 patients. Aulitzky and coworkers [2] showed that a relatively low dose of γ-IFN, 100 μg (2×10^6 IU) once weekly, was biologically more active than higher doses. The low dose resulted in a nearly maximal rise of neopterin and β_2-microglobulin levels in the serum with minimal side effects, whereby the increments in these markers were predictive for response.

Clinical trials with α-IFN monotherapy showed modest, but reproducible antitumor activity in RCC; pooled data indicated a response rate of 15% [21, 26]. Results with γ-IFN monotherapy are disappointing. Garnick et al. found a response rate of 9.7% [17], while two other studies showed no responses [29, 31]. Otto et al., however, observed a total of five responders in a small series of 16 patients (31%) [28]. In all three model systems, clonogenic assay, nude mice and rats, we could show that combinations of BRM have synergistic antiproliferative effects. In clinical trials too, combination treatment is more effective than monotherapy. Low-dose combination treatment with α-IFN and γ-IFN resulted in a 28% rate of objective responses [18].

Combinations of IFN and TNF which were very effective when treatment was started within 48 h after tumor implantation did not inhibit tumor growth when started at higher tumor volumes [39]. The combination of the highest doses of IFN and TNF, however, significantly inhibited tumor growth, although it did not induce tumor regression. A similar influence of tumor volume at start of therapy was elegantly shown for experimental prostatic carcinoma [20]. These experiments clearly demonstrated the need for tumor debulking and adjuvant chemotherapy as early as possible in order to minimize the total tumor load and maximize the possibility of cure. Our studies, therefore, imply that patients with RCC might benefit most from immunotherapy when this treatment is started as early as possible, i.e., in the case of localized disease, immediately after nephrectomy. Side effects of cytokine treatments, however, force us to select patients at risk for clinical progression. The lack of good inclusion criteria for adjuvant immunotherapy protocols may hamper the start of such trails.

Questions with regard to treatment schedule and BRM choice in RCC remain unanswered. Sequential treatment could be a good alternative. Pretreatment of tumor cells with IFN, for example, can enhance or induce the sensitivity of cells for TNF [24] in vitro. Other BRMs and their combinations have to be tested. In animal models, triple combination therapy with TNF, IL-2 and alpha-IFN improved therapeutic results and reduced toxicity [27].

The combination of chemotherapy with immunotherapy seems very promising. IFN synergistically potentiates the activity of a wide variety of cytotoxic agents against multiple rodent and human tumors [41]. Another potentially therapeutic combination is that of TNF with drugs targeted against DNA topoisomerase II, such as Adriamycin, actinomycin D and VP-16 [1]. The combination of VP-16 and TNF given after nephrectomy resulted in a significant decrease in local recurrence and no evidence of metastasis in an animal model study [7]. In the syngeneic rat renal cell tumor we found synergistic antiproliferative effects of TNF in combination with various doses of Adriamycin in vitro; in vivo studies, however, showed modest synergistic effects only with combinations including the highest dose of Adriamycin.

Passive immunotherapy with monoclonal antibodies has been hampered by the lack of tumor-specific reagents. Recently an anti-RCC monoclonal antibody (MAb), G250, was described which recognizes an antigen present on RCC but not on normal cells. Bispecific MAb were developed by somatic hybridization of two mouse hybridomas, one producing MAb against G250 RCC-associated antigen and the other against T-cell antigen CD3 (OKT3) [38]. The dual specificity of the hybrid MAb produced by these so-called quadromas was analyzed in vitro. The bispecific MAb induced T cells to kill RCC cells. The bispecific MAb bridge the effector cells (cytotoxic T cells) and the target cells. The high specificity of G250 for RCC and the high levels of specific cell lysis obtained at low concentrations of bispecific MAb suggest that these MAb can be of therapeutic value in RCC. First in vivo experiments showed that combinations of peripheral blood lymphocytes and bispecific MAb neutralized tumor growth of the TK82 xenograft [25]. Since both cytokines and MAb have their specific effects on the immune system, combination of these treatment modalities might enhance their effects. Experiments to test this hypothesis are currently under way.

Rational design of new treatment protocols is hampered by the lack of fundamental understanding of the mechanism of action of BRMs. Therefore, more preclinical studies are urgently needed to develop effective systemic therapies against disseminated RCC.

References

1. Alexander RB, Nelson WG, Coffey DS (1987) Synergistic enhancement by tumor necrosis factor of in vitro cytotoxicity from chemotherapeutic drugs targeted at DNA topoisomerase II. Cancer Res 47:2403
2. Aulitzky W, Gastl G, Aulitzky WE, Herold M, Kemmler J, Mull B, Frick J, Huber Ch (1989) Successful treatment of metastatic renal cell carcinoma with a biologically active dose of recombinant interferon-gamma. J Clin Oncol 7:1875
3. Balkwill FR, Lee A, Aldam G, Moodie E, Thomas JA, Tavernier J, Fiers W (1987) Human tumor xenografts treated with recombinant human tumor necrosis factor alone or in combination with interferons. Cancer Res 46:3990
4. Belldegrun A, Muul LM, Rosenberg SA (1988) Interleukin-2 expanded tumor-infiltrating lymphocytes in human renal cell cancer: isolation, characterization, and antitumor activity. Cancer Res 48:206
5. Beniers AJMC, van Moorselaar RJA, Peelen WP, Hendriks BTh, Otto U, Schalken JA, Debruyne FMJ (1989) In vitro sensitivity of three human renal tumor xenografts towards tumor necrosis factor and alpha and gamma interferon. In: Rübben H, Jocham D, Jacobi GH (eds) Investigative urology 3. Springer, Berlin Heidelberg New York, pp 30–38
6. Beniers AJMC, van Moorselaar RJA, Peelen WP, Debruyne FMJ, Schalken JA (1990) Tumor growth inhibition of renal cell carcinoma xenografts after therapy with interferon and tumor necrosis factor (in press)
7. Burgers JK, Marshall FF, Isaacs JT (1989) Enhanced anti-tumor effects of recombinant human tumor necrosis factor plus VP-16 on metastatic renal cell carcinoma in a xenograft model. J Urol 142:160
8. Carswell EA, Old LJ, Kassel RL, Green S, Fiore N, Williamson B (1975) An endotoxin-induced serum factor that causes necrosis of tumors. Proc Natl Acad Sci USA 72:3666
9. Czarniecki CW, Christopher WF, Powers DV, Estell DA (1984) Synergistic antiviral and antiproliferative activities of *E. coli*-derived human alpha, beta and gamma interferons. J Virol 49:490
10. deKernion JB, Mukamel E (1987) Selection of initial therapy for renal cell carcinoma. Cancer 60:539
11. Droller MJ (1986) Immunotherapy and genitourinary neoplasia: an overview. World J Urol 3:200
12. Feitz WFJ, Verheyen RHM, Kirkels WJ, Vooijs GP, Debruyne FMJ, Herman CJ (1986) Dynamics of human renal tumor colony growth in vitro. Urol Res 14:109
13. Fisher RI, Coltman CA, Doroshow JH, Rayner AA, Hawkins MJ, Mier JW, Wiernik P et al. (1988) Metastatic renal cancer treated with interleukin-2 and lymphokine-activated killer cells. A phase II clinical trial. Ann Intern Med 108:518
14. Foon KA (1989) Biological response modifiers: the new immunotherapy. Cancer Res 49:1621
15. Fransen L, van der Heyden J, Ruysscchaert R, Fiers W (1986) Recombinant tumor necrosis factor: its effect and its synergism with interferon-gamma on a variety of normal and transformed human cell lines. Eur J Cancer Clin Oncol 22:419
16. Freed SZ, Halperin JP, Gordon M (1977) Idiopathic regression of metastases from renal cell carcinoma. J Urol 118:538
17. Garnick MB, Reich SD, Maxwell B, Coval-Goldsmith S, Richie JP, Rudnick SA (1988) Phase I/II study of recombinant interferon-gamma in advanced renal cell carcinoma. J Urol 139:251
18. Geboers ADH, de Mulder PHM, Debruyne FMJ, Strijk SP, Damsma O (1988) Alpha and gamma interferon in the treatment of advanced renal cell carcinoma. Sem Surg Oncol 4:191

19. Harris DT (1983) Hormonal therapy and chemotherapy of renal-cell carcinoma. Semin Oncol 10:422
20. Henry JM, Isaacs JT (1988) Relationship between tumor size and the curability of metastatic prostatic cancer by surgery alone or in combination with adjuvant chemotherapy. J Urol 139:1119
21. Horoszewicz JS, Murphy GP (1989) An assessment of the current use of human interferons in therapy of urological tumors. J Urol 142:1173–1180
22. Hubbel HR, Craft JA, Leibowitz PJ, Gillespie DH (1987) Synergistic antiproliferative effect of recombinant alpha-interferons with recombinant interferon-gamma. J Biol Resp Mod 6:141
23. Karthaus HFM, Feitz WFJ, van der Meijden APM, Schalken JA, Beck JLM, Hendriks BTh, Jap PHK et al. (1987) Multidisciplinary evaluation of rat renal cell carcinoma. In vivo 1:335
24. Kavoussi LR, Ruesing RA, Hudson MA, Catalona WJ, Ratliff TL (1989) Effect of tumor necrosis factor and interferon gamma on human renal carcinoma cell line growth. J Urol 142:875
25. Kerr LA, Huntoon CJ, Nelson H, Leibson PJ, Segal D, Donohue JH, Vessella R et al. (1990) Immunotherapy of renal cell carcinoma using the G250/OKT3 bispecific antibody. J Urol 143:321A
26. Krown SE (1987) Interferon treatment of renal cell carcinoma. Current status and future prospects. Cancer 59:647
27. McIntosh JK, Mulé JJ, Krosnick JA, Rosenberg SA (1989) Combination cytokine immunotherapy with tumor necrosis factor alpha, interleukin 2, and alpha-interferon and its synergistic antitumor effects in mice. Cancer Res 49:1408
28. Otto U, Conrad S, Schneider AW (1988) Recombinant interferon-gamma in the treatment of metastatic RCC. Arzneim Forsch/Drug Res 38:1658
29. Quesada JR, Kurzrock R, Sherwin SA, Gutterman JU (1987) Phase II studies of recombinant interferon gamma in metastatic renal cell carcinoma. J Biol Resp Mod 6:20
30. Rauschmeier HA (1988) Immunotherapy of metastatic renal cancer. Semin Surg Oncol 4:169
31. Rinehart JJ, Malspeis L, Young D, Neidthart JA (1986) Phase I-II trial of recombinant interferon gamma in renal cell carcinoma. J Biol Resp Mod 5:300
32. Rosenberg SA, Lotze MT, Muul LM, Chang AE, Avis FP, Leitman S, Linehan WM et al. (1987) A progress report on the treatment of 157 patients with advanced cancer using lymphokine-activated killer cells and interleukin-2 or high-dose interleukin-2 alone. N Engl J Med 316:889
33. Shah P, van der Meide PH, Borman T, Schroeder N, Bliss JM, Coombes RC (1989) Effect of human recombinant tumour necrosis factor and rat gamma interferon on nitrosomethylurea-induced mammary tumors. Br J Cancer 59:206
34. Silverberg S (1987) Statistical and epidemiologic data on urologic cancer. Cancer 60:692
35. Strander H (1986) Interferon treatment in human neoplasia. Adv Cancer Res 46:10
36. Sugarman BJ, Aggarwal BB, Hass PE, Figari IS, Palladino MA, Shepard HM (1985) Recombinant human tumor necrosis factor-alpha: effects on proliferation of normal and transformed cells in vitro. Science 230:943
37. Talmadge JE, Tribble HR, Pennington RW, Phillips H, Wiltrout RH (1987) Immunomodulatory and immunotherapeutic properties of recombinant gamma-interferon and recombinant tumor necrosis factor alpha in mice. Cancer Res 47:2563
38. van Dijk J, Warnaar SO, van Eendenburg JDH, Thienpont M, Braakman E, Boot JHA, Fleuren JH, Bolhuis RLH (1989) Induction of tumor-cell lysis by bi-specific monoclonal antibodies recognizing renal-cell carcinoma and CD3 antigen. Int J Cancer 43:344

39. van Moorselaar RJA, Beniers AJMC, Hendriks BTh, van der Meide PH, Schellekens H, Debruyne FMJ, Schalken JA (1990) In vivo antiproliferative effects of gamma-interferon and tumor necrosis factor alpha in a rat renal cell carcinoma model system. J Urol 143:1247
40. van Moorselaar RJA, Beniers AJMC, Hendriks BTh, Debruyne FMJ, Schalken JA (1990) Antiproliferative effects of adriamycin and tumor necrosis factor alpha in a rat renal cell tumor model system. J Urol 143:387A
41. Wadler S, Schwartz EL (1990) Antineoplastic activity of the combination of interferon and cytotoxic agents against experimental and human malignancies: a review. Cancer Res 50:3473

Clinical Experience with Biological Response Modifiers in Renal Cell Carcinoma

Rationale for Immunotherapy in Renal Cell Carcinoma

R. Heicappell and R. Ackermann[1]

The majority of deaths from human cancers are due to the fact that tumor cells detach from the primary tumor and settle in distant organs to form metastases. In renal cell carcinoma (RCC), approximately 50% of the patients who present with initial symptoms will succumb to distant metastases in the course of their disease. Some 80% of the patients with disseminated disease will die within 3 years after surgery whereas 65% of patients with localized disease survive at least 5 years after diagnosis [7].

As in other types of disseminated cancer, attempts at therapy of disseminated RCC have been based on three traditional approaches: surgery [9], chemotherapy [39], and radiotherapy [2, 29]. None of them has significantly improved the prognosis of patients with disseminated disease.

The failure of chemotherapy for disseminated RCC could possibly be due to the expression of the multidrug resistance (MDR) gene that has been demonstrated in 80% of human RCC [12]. The MDR gene codes for a 170 000-dalton glycoprotein (P-glycoprotein) that serves as a transmembrane efflux pump for cytotoxic drugs and thereby makes chemotherapy ineffective in a variety of cancers [20]. The reasons for failure of surgery and radiotherapy in the treatment of RCC are unknown at present. Thus, there is no commonly accepted therapy available for metastatic RCC. Instead, therapy of advanced RCC is a challenge for new therapeutic approaches because there is virtually no alternative.

Observations of spontaneous regression of RCC metastases have led to the concept that the disappearance of distant metastases without therapy may be due to rejection of the metastases by the immune system. Spontaneous regression of RCC metastases is a rare event with a frequency of approximately 0.5% [8]. So far, no direct evidence has been presented for involvement of the immune system in the rejection of tumor metastases in humans.

Attempts at immunotherapy of advanced RCC have been made for more than 15 years ago (for review see [22, 23]). Most of them employed nonspecific immunostimulators and/or relatively crude preparations of mediators with immunostimulatory activity. In the meantime, major advances in immunology and molecular biology have brought about a variety of new drugs and therapeutic approaches with potential antiproliferative and/or cytotoxic activities which are being used in

[1] Urologische Klinik der Universität, Moorenstr. 5, W–4000 Düsseldorf 1, FRG

F.M.J. Debruyne et al. (Eds.)
Immunotherapy of Renal Cell Carcinoma

clinical phase I and phase II trials. Most recent clinical trials for immunotherapy of advanced RCC focus on three major approaches (for review see [10, 16, 27]):

1) active specific immunotherapy,
2) recombinant cytokines, and
3) adoptive transfer of immunocompetent cells.

The first two, either alone or in combination with adoptive transfer of immunocompetent cells, have been used in clinical trails.

The initial step in immune responses is recognition of a structure on the target cell, the antigen. Most antigens in RCC have been demonstrated serologically. Several groups have raised murine monoclonal antibodies against human RCC. With a few exceptions [26, 33], serologically defined antigens in h-RCC are not exclusively found on cancer cells; they are also seen on nontransformed renal cells, particularly on tubular epithelium cells (for review see [3]). Antigens that are expressed on normal renal cells may be modulated in renal cancer [6]. Other antigens found in RCC include receptors for hormones like that for vitamin 1,25 D_3 [24]. Moreover, several leukocyte differentiation antigens have been demonstrated in human RCCs [4].

Serologically defined antigens (e.g., by monoclonal or polyclonal antibodies) in h-RCC have been used as targets for immunolocalization and monoclonal antibody-targeted radiotherapy in experimental animals (for review see [15]). Monoclonal antibodies with specificity for the tumor antigen and the antigen receptor of cytoxic T cells have been shown to enhance T-cell mediated cytolysis greatly both in vitro [37] and in nude mice [38].

Whereas monoclonal antibodies have been used in the therapy of leukemias, lymphomas, gastrointestinal tract tumors, and melanoma (for review see [13]), phase II studies with monoclonal antibodies have not been reported with RCC.

T lymphocytes may lyse tumor cells after recognition and very specific binding. The antigens that are recognized by tumor-specific T lymphocytes are poorly defined as yet. Nevertheless, attempts have been made to immunize patients against their own tumor in order to elicit tumor rejection. Clinical trials have been set up with different kinds of tumor vaccines [14, 25, 31, 32, 35]. Vaccines for immunization against tumors usually contain tumor antigen plus more or less defined adjuvants like bacteria or viruses. Heicappell et al. have presented evidence that by addition of a nonpathogenic paramyxovirus to tumor vaccines tumor-specific T-cell responses can be augmented considerably in mouse tumors [17]. Results of clinical trials for immunization against RCC are conflicting, with objective responses ranging between 0% and 25%. Most likely, these differences are due to patient selection and the lack of knowledge of the exact mechanism of T-cell-mediated tumor rejection. Currently, the role of tumor antigen and T lymphocytes in tumor rejection is being investigated [1, 11, 17, 34].

Tumor rejection by the immune system is not exclusively mediated by cellular elements of the immune system. Rather, soluble molecules secreted by immune cells (e.g., lymphocytes, macrophages, natural killer cells) have been discovered that play an important role in tumor rejection. These molecules have been termed cytokines. Some cytokines have been shown to possess direct cytotoxicity towards human tumor cells (e.g., tumor necrosis factor), some are growth inhibitory but not cytotoxic (e.g., interferon alpha, IFNα), some do not have direct effects on tumor cells at all (e.g., interleukin-2, IL-2), and some do not even interfere with tumor growth (granulocyte macrophage colony stimulating factor).

Cytokines have several features in common. Typically, recombinant cytokines have molecular weights in the range of 15–40 kD. In vivo, they usually possess a short half-life only. Thus, in order to maintain effective levels systemically, high doses of the respective cytokines have to be infused. Therapy with cytokines usually has typical and sometimes severe side effects.

Interferons, more specifically IFNα have been used for therapy of RCC in many clinical trials (for review see [18]). Consistently, a 15% rate for objective responses to therapy with IFNα has been reported. IFNβ or IFNγ were of marginal activity only.

IL-2 serves as a growth factor for activated T lymphocytes. Moreover, Rosenberg and coworkers have observed that a certain subpopulation of T-lymphocytes may be rendered cytolytic for fresh tumor cells in a nonspecific way by addition of IL-2. The lymphocytes have been termed lymphokine-activated killer (LAK) cells. Consequently, clinical trials have been set up with IL-2 and LAK cells. T lymphocytes from the peripheral blood or tumor-infiltrating lymphocytes have been activated in vitro with IL-2 and reinfused into the patients after expansion in IL-2. This approach yields approximately 20%–30% objective responses, with even long-term survivors [21, 30].

IL-2/LAK cell therapy is hampered by severe and sometimes life-threatening side effects. Attempts have been made to reduce this toxicity, and the handling of LAK cells is restricted to specialized centers. In this respect, a regimen with continuous infusion of IL-2 without transfusion of LAK cells has been tried and yielded comparable results to trials with both IL-2 and LAK cells [36]. Moreover, IL-2 has been applied in combination with chemotherapeutic drugs and other cytokines. Ancouraging results (approx. 20%–25% objective response) have been reported, specifically from clinical trials that combines IL-2 with IFNα (Bukowski 1989) or IFNβ (Krigel 1989).

From the data briefly summarized here it can be concluded that there clearly is a rationale for immunotherapy of RCC. Immunotherapy is a new and still experimental approach for the treatment of metastases. Knowledge of the immune system and its regulation is steadily increasing. Thus, it can be expected that new and improved regimens will be developed in the near future.

References

1. Bianchi R, Romani L, Puccetti P, Fioretti M (1988) Induction of tumor suppression and delayed-type footpad reaction by transfer of lymphocytes sensitized to a xenogenized tumor variant. Int J Cancer 42:71–75
2. Brady LW (1983) Carcinoma of the kidney – role of radiotherapy. Sem Oncol 10 (4):417–421
3. Bander NH (1989) Monoclonal antibodies to renal cancer antigens. Sem Urol 7 (4):264–270
4. Borowitz MJ, Weiss MA, Bossen EH, Metzger R (1986) Characterization of renal neoplasms with monoclonal antibodies to leukocyte differentiation antigens. Cancer 57 (2):251–256
5. Bukowski RM, Goodman P, Crawford ED, Sergi JS, Baker L, Neidhart J (1989) Phase II evaluation of recombinant interleukin-2 (RIL-2) in metastatic renal cell carcinoma (RCC): SWOG 8617. Proc Am Soc Clin Oncol 8:A556
6. Cordon-Cardo C, Reuter VE, Finstad CL, Sheinfeld J, Lloyd KO, Fair WR, Melamed MR (1989) Blood group-related antigens in human kidney: modulation of Lewis determinants in renal cell carcinoma. Cancer Res 49 (1):212–218
7. deKernion JB, Ramming KP, Smith RB (1978) The natural history of metastatic renal cell carcinoma: a computer analysis. J Urol 120:148–152
8. deKernion JB, Berry D (1980) The diagnosis and treatment of renal cell carcinoma. Cancer 45:1947–1956
9. Dineen MK, Pastore RD, Emrich LJ, Huben RP (1988) Results of surgical treatment of renal cell carcinoma with solitary metastasis. J Urol 140:277–279
10. Droller MJ (1987) Biologic response modifiers in genitourinary neoplasia. Cancer 60 (Suppl):635–644
11. Fearon ER, Itaya T, Hunt B, Vogelstein B, Frost P (1988) Induction of immunogenic tumor variants by transfection with an foreign gene. Cancer Research 48:2975–2980
12. Fojo AT, Shen D-W, Mickley LA, Pastan IA, Gottesman MM (1987) Intrinsic drug resistance in human kidney cancer is associated with expression of a human multidrug resistance gene. J Clin Oncol 5 (12):1922–1927
13. Foon KA (1989) Biological response modifiers: the new immunotherapy. Cancer Res 49:1621–1639
14. Fowler JE Jr (1986) Failure of immunotherapy for metastatic renal cell carcinoma. J Urol 135:22–25
15. Fritzberg AR (1989) Antibody targeted radiotherapy. Proc Am Ass Cancer Res 30:648
16. Graham SD (1989) Immunotherapy of renal cell carcinoma. Sem Urol 7 (4):215–227
17. Heicappell R, Schirrmacher V, von Hoegen P, Ahlert P, Appelhans B (1986) Prevention of postoperative metastatic spread by postoperative immunotherapy with virally modified autologous tumor cells. I. Parameters for optimal therapeutic effect. Int J Cancer 37:569–577
18. Horoszewicz JS, Murphy GP (1989) An assessment of the current use of human interferons in therapy of urological cancer. J Urol 142:1173–1180
19. Krigel R, Padavic K, Rudolph A, Comis R (1988) Phase II study of recombinant interleukin-2 (RIL-2) plus recombinant beta interferon (IFN-beta) in advanced renal cell carcinoma. Proc Am Soc Clin Oncol 7:A509
20. Ling V, Kartner N, Sudo T, Siminovitch L, Riordan JR (1983) Multidrug resistance phenotype in chinese hamster ovary cells. Cancer Treatm Report 67:869–874
21. Margolin KA, Rayner AA, Hawkins MJ, Atkins MB, Butcher JP, Fisher RI, Weiss GR et al. (1989) Interleukin2 and lymphokine-activated killer cell therapy of solid tumors: analysis of toxocity and management guidelines. J Clin Oncol 7 (4):486–498
22. McCune CS (1983) Immunologic therapies of kidney carcinoma. Sem Oncol 10 (4):431–436

23. Montie JE, Bukowski RM, Lee RJ, Straffon RA, Stewart BH (1982) A critical review of immunotherapy of disseminated renal adenocarcinoma. J Surg Oncol 21:5–8
24. Nagakura K, Hayakawa M, Hata M, Nakamura H (1987) 1,25-Dihydroxyvitamin D_3 receptors and their relationship to histological features in renal cell carcinoma. J Urol 137:1300–1303
25. Neidhardt JA, Murphy SG, Hennick LA, Wise HA (1980) Active specific immunotherapy of stage IV renal carcinoma with aggregated tumor antigen adjuvant. Cancer 46:1128–1139
26. Oosterwijk E, Ruiter DJ, Hoedemaker PJ, Pauwels EK, Jonas U, Zwartendijk J, Warnaar SO (1986) Monoclonal antibody G 250 recognizes a determinant present in renal cell carcinoma and absent from normal kidney. Int J Cancer 38:489
27. Quesada J (1988) Biologic response modifiers in the therapy of metastatic renal cell carcinoma. Sem Oncol 15 (4):396–407
28. Rieden K, Adolph J, Lellig U, zum Winkel K (1989) Strahlentherapeutischer Effekt bei Knochenmetastasen in Abhängigkeit von der Metastasenhäufigkeit, Metastasenlokalisation und der Histologie des Primärtumors. Strahlenther Onkol 165 (5):P380–385
29. Rosenberg SE, Spiess P, Lanafriere R (1986) A new approach to the adoptive immunotherapy of cancer with tumor-infiltrating lymphocytes. Science 233:1318–1321
30. Rosenberg SE, Lotze MT, Muul LM, Chang AE, Avis FP, Leitman S, Marston Linehan W et al. (1987) A progress report on the treatment of 157 patiens with advanced cancer using lymphocine-activated killer cells and interleukin-2 or high dose interleukin-2 alone. N Engl J Med 316:889–905
31. Sahasrabudhe DM, deKornion JB, Pontes JE, Ryan DM, O'Donnell RW, Marwuis DM, Mudholkar GS, McCune CS (1986) Specific immunotherapy with suppressor function inhibition of metastatic renal cell carcinoma. J Biol Resp Mod 5 (6):581–594
32. Schärfe T, Klippel KF, Jacobi GH, Hohenfellner R (1983) Tumor specific immunotherapy for metastatic renal cell carcinoma (meeting abstract). 78th Annual Meeting of the American Urological Association
33. Schärfe T, Störkel St, Yokohama M, Kaltwasser R, Thüroff J, Jacobi GH, Hohenfellner R (1988) Tumor-specific antigen for human renal cell carcinoma. Eur Urol 14:464–469
34. Schirrmacher V, Fogel M, Russmann E, Bosslet K, Altevogt P, Beck L (1982) Antigenic variation in cancer metastasis: immune escape versus immune control. Cancer Metastasis Reviews 1:241–274
35. Tallberg T, Tykkä H (1986) Specific active immunotherapy in advanced renal cell carcinoma: a clinical longterm follow-up study. World J Urol 3:234–244
36. Thompson JA, Lee DL, Lindgren CG, Benz LA, Collins C, Levitt D, Fefer A (1988) Influence of dose and duration of infusion on interleukin-2 on toxicity and immunomodulation. J Clin Oncol 6 (4):669–678
37. van Dijk J, Warnaar SO, van Eendenburg JDH, Thienpont M, Braakman E, Boot JHA, Fleuren GJ, Bildhuis RHL (1989) Induction of tumor cell lysis by bi-specific monoclonal antibodies recognizing renal-cell carcinoma and CD3 antigen. Int J Cancer 43:344–349
38. Wunderlich JR, Garrido MA, Valdayo M, Winkler DF, Titus JA, Perez P, Qian J, Segal DM (1989) Targeting human T cells with bispecific antibodies to react with human tumors growing in immunodeficient mice. Proc Am Ass Cancer Res 30:647
39. Yagoda A (1989) Chemotherapy of renal cell carcinoma. Sem Urol 7 (4):199–206

Treatment of Renal Cell Carcinoma with Interferon

M.P. Wirth[1]

The successful use of interferon-α (IFN-α) in the treatment of metastasized renal cell carcinoma (RCC) was first reported in 1983 [5]. Since that time the efficacy of IFN-α in RCC has been tested in numerous studies. Recently the two other IFN, namely IFN-β and IFN-γ, have also been used in the treatment of RCC. Although we know much more about the subtypes and the action of IFN today than we did in 1983, the exact mechanisms of tumor control by IFN have not yet been elucidated.

Interferons generally can act as antiproliferative agents. In addition they have antiviral and immunomodulating activities and they inhibit oncogene expression in tumor cells. However, IFN-γ differs from IFN-α and IFN-β regarding the immuneregulating activity.

Interferon-α

Interferon-α has been utilized in the vast majority of the studies. The first responses of RCC were observed when crude leukocyte IFN was used. The results were subsequently reproduced with highly purified human lymphoblastoid IFN-α and with purified recombinant IFN-α. IFN-α produces an overall objective response rate of 16%. This is in the same range as lymphoblastoid IFN (13%) and the recombinant IFN-α2a and IFN-α2b (14%) [8]. The data summarized in Table 1 demonstrate that the recombinant IFN-α2a and -α2b, which each consist of only one of the 21 subtypes of natural IFN-α, act in the same way as natural IFN-α. The response rates have varied among studies, probably owing to differences in treatment regimen, dosage, selection of patients and other unknown factors. Patient selection is the most important factor regarding response rates. In patients with metastases to the lungs only and a good performance status, response rates of 40% can be achieved using IFN-α. Interferon-α shows almost no activity, however, against bone, brain and liver metastases. Regarding the optimal dosage of IFN-α, it was demonstrated in randomized trials by Quesada and co-workers [14] and by Kirkwood et al. [6] that there is a positive relationship between dosage and response. This may suggest that the action of IFN-α is at least partly antiproliferative, since immunostimulation occurs also if low doses of IFN are administered. High doses of IFN, however,

[1] Department of Urology, University of Würzburg, Medical School, W–8700 Würzburg, FRG

F.M.J. Debruyne et al. (Eds.)
Immunotherapy of Renal Cell Carcinoma

cause severe side effects. For this reason Krown [8] divided IFN dosing into three categories: low doses which induce minimal toxicity, intermediate doses which leads to moderate toxicity and high doses which cause severe dose-limiting toxicities in more than 50% of the patients. For human leukocyte IFN-α the intermediate doserange is 3–6 million units per day. For recombinant IFN-α2a and IFN-α2b and for lymphoblastoid IFN-α, 5–20 million units per day is considered intermediate. Low doses are ineffective, but intermediate dosages of IFN-α result in the best overall response rates, namely 19%, as summarized by Krown in 1987 [8]. High, toxic doses lead to markedly decreased response rates. The mean time to response with IFN-α is about 3 months, and the mean duration of response is between 5 and 15 months (Table 2). Regarding treatment schedules, significant and similar responses have been observed giving IFN-α 7 days a week, 5 days a week or in cycles of 5–10 days of treatment every 2–3 weeks. However, the optimal dose and administration schedule for IFN-α have not been defined so far.

Interferon-β

Data on the use of IFN-β in RCC are sparse. In 1986, Rinehart and co-workers [15] reported partial responses in two of 15 patients treated with recombinant IFN-β.

Table 1. Results of treatment with different types of IFN-α in renal cell cancer

Reference	Authors	Year	IFN-α	*n*	Dose (Mill/U)	Response rate (CR + PR, %)
[5]	deKernion et al.	1983	LE	43	3	16
[15]	Quesada et al.	1985	LE	50		26
[1]	Edsmyr et al.	1985	LE	11	3	27
[6]	Kirkwood et al.	1985	LE	14	1	0
			LE	16	10	18
[14]	Quesada et al.	1985	re-α2a	41	20	29
				15	2	0
[18]	Umeda et al.	1986	re-α2a	108	3–36	14
[17]	Sarna et al.	1987	re-α2a	24	3–36	26
[18]	Umeda et al.	1986	re-α2b	45	3–36	20
[9]	Muss et al.	1987	re-α2b	51	30	7
[19]	Vugrin et al.	1985	Ly	21	3	5
[18]	Umeda et al.	1986	Ly	93	5	23

LE, Leukocyte IFN-α; *re*, recombinant IFN-α; *Ly*, lymphoblastoid IFN-α

Table 2. Characteristics of response to IFN

Reference	Authors	Year	IFN	Mean time to response in months (range)	Mean duration of response in months (range)
[10]	Neidhart et al.	1984	IFN-α-N1 (low dose)	3.0 (0.6–6.3)	5 (5–10)
[15]	Quesada et al.	1985	HuIFN-2 (LE)	3.0 (1.0–7.0)	7 (2–16)
[11]	Neidhart et al.	1984	IFN-α-N1 (high dose)	2.2 (2.0–30)	15 (2–36)
[2]	Fujita et al.	1988	IFN-α-N1	3.0 (1.0–8.0)	6.5 (1–20)

Table 3. Results of IFN-γ treatment in patients with metastatic renal cell carcinoma

Reference	Authors	Year	*n*	Responses (CR + PR) *n*	%
[14]	Quesada et al.	1985	30	2	7
[7]	Koiso et al.	1987	62	8	13
[3]	Garnick et al.	1988	42	4	9.7
[4]	Huber et al.	1988	16	8	50
[12]	Otto et al.	1988	16	5	32
	Dept. of Urology, Univ. of Würzburg	1989	10	3	30

Interferon-γ

The results of IFN-γ treatment of metastatic RCC reported in the literature, including our own, differ widely. One reason for this could be the different treatment regimens applied. Response rates range from less than 10% to 50% (Table 3). It is unclear as yet whether optimal immunostimulation is responsible for the excellent results – objective response rates of 50% – claimed by Huber and associates [4] on giving IFN-γ once a week. However, the greater immunomodulatory potency of IFN-γ, compared with IFN-α and IFN-β, may play a role. This greater potency includes activation of macrophages, enhancement of antibody-dependent cellular cytotoxicity, enhancement of Fc receptors, enhancement of HLA DR antigens and functional interaction with interleukin-2.

Conclusions

Interferon-α monotherapy in metastasized RCC leads to overall response rates of only about 19% if optimal doses are used. The response rates reported for IFN-γ range widely, from less than 10% to 50%. Optimal dosages and intervals have not yet been defined. The low overall response rates of monotherapy using IFN-α or IFN-γ in larger series are disappointing. Additional forms of treatment for metastasized RCC are urgently needed.

References

1. Edsmyr F, Esposti PL, Andersson L, Steineck G, Lagergren C, Strander H (1985) Interferon therapy in disseminated renal cell carcinoma. Radiother Oncol 4:21–26
2. Fujita T, Asano H, Naide Y, Ono Y, Onshima S, Suzuki K, Aso Y et al. (1988) Antitumor effects of human lymphoblastoid interferon on advanced renal cell carcinoma. J Urol 139:256–258
3. Garnick MB, Reich SD, Maxwell B, Coval-Goldsmith S, Richie JP, Rudnick SA (1988) Phase I/II study of recombinant interferon gamma in advanced renal cell carcinoma. J Urol 139:251–255
4. Huber C, Aulitzky W, Gastl G, Aulitzky WE, Herold M, Frick J (1989) Treatment of metastasizing renal cell carcinoma with an optimum biological response modifying dose of r-IFN-gamma. J Biol Resp Mod 8:335
5. deKernion JB, Sarna JB, Figlin R, Lindner A, Smith RB (1983) The treatment of renal cell carcinoma with human leukocyte alpha-interferon. J Urol 130:1063–1066
6. Kirkwood JM, Harris JE; Vera R, Sandler S, Fischer DS, Khandekar J, Ernstoff MS et al. (1985) A randomized study of low and high doses of leukocyte alpha-interferon in metastatic renal cell carcinoma: the American Cancer Society collaborative trial. Cancer Res 45:863–871
7. Koiso K and Recombinant Human Interferon Gamma (S-6810) Research Group on Renal Cell Carcinoma (1987) Phase II study of recombinant human interferon gamma (S-6810) on renal cell carcinoma. Cancer 60:929–933
8. Krown SE (1987) Interferon treatment of renal cell carcinoma. Current status and future prospects. Cancer 59:647–651
9. Muss HB, Constanzi JJ, Leavitt R, Williams RD, Kempf RA, Pollard R, Ozer H et al. (1987) Recombinant alpha interferon in renal cell carcinoma: a randomized trial of two routes of administration. J Clin Oncol 5:286–291
10. Neidhart JA, Gagen MM, Young D, Tuttle R, Melink TJ, Ziccarrelli A, Kisner D (1984) Interferon-alpha therapy of renal cancer. Cancer Res 44:4140–4143
11. Neidhart J, Gagen M, Kisner R, Tuttel R, Whisman J (1984) Therapy of renal cancer with low (LD) and high (HD) dose regimens of human lymphoblastoid interferon (HBLJ; Wellferon). Proc Am Soc Clin Oncol 3:60
12. Otto U, Schneider A, Denkhaus H, Conrad S (1988) Die Behandlung des metastasierten Nierenkarzinoms mit rekombinantem alpha-2- oder gamma-Interferon. Ergebnisse zweier klinischer Phase-II- bzw. -III-Studien. Onkologie 11:185–191
13. Quesada JR, Swanson DA, Trindade A, Gutterman JU (1983) Renal cell carcinoma: Antitumor effects of leukocyte interferon. Cancer Res 43:940–947
14. Quesada JR, Rios A, Swanson D, Trown P, Gutterman JU (1985) Antitumor activity of recombinant-derived interferon alpha in metastatic renal cell carcinoma. J Clin Oncol 3:1522–1528

15. Quesada JR, Swanson DA, Gutterman JU (1985) Phase II study of interferon alpha in metastatic renal cell carcinoma. J Clin Oncol 3:1086–1092
16. Rinehart J, Malspeis L, Young D, Neidhart J (1986) Phase I/II trial of human recombinant beta-interferon serine in patients with renal cell carcinoma. Cancer Res 46:5364–5367
17. Sarna G, Figlin R, deKernion J (1987) Interferon in renal cell carcinoma. The UCLA experience. Cancer 59:610–612
18. Umeda T, Niijima T (1986) Phase II study of alpha-interferon on renal cell carcinoma. Summary of three collaborative trials. Cancer 58:1231–1235
19. Vugrin D, Hood L, Taylor W, Laszlo J (1985) Phase II study of human lymphoblastoid interferon in patients with advanced renal carcinoma. Cancer Treat Rep 69:817–820

Combination Therapy with Interferon in Renal Cell Carcinoma

S.D. Fosså[1]

Introduction

Interferon alpha (IFNα) yields a 15%–20% response rate in patients with metastatic renal cell carcinoma (RCC) when given as monotherapy at doses of 9–18 $\times$ 10^6 U thrice weekly [22]. There seems to be no significant difference in the response rates obtained by different IFNs: IFNα, IFNβ, natural leukocyte IFN, or recombinant IFN. Monotherapy with IFNγ has, however, been insufficiently evaluated in clinical studies. Due to the considerable interstudy variability of the selection criteria of patients treated with IFN, the overall role of this drug in the management of metastatic RCC cannot yet be determined. However, IFN therapy of RCC represents the first treatment of this malignancy which has consistently achieved a response rate of 10% or more. The most frequently responding sites are lung metastases [27]. Treatment should be given for at least 2 months unless the patient progresses before this time interval has elapsed. Patients who after 2 months show an at least 30% reduction have a reasonable chance of finally obtaining an objective response [15]. Responders usually live longer than nonresponders [4, 15], which, however, may mirror a biologically less aggressive disease rather than treatment efficacy.

Flulike symptoms (fever, muscle pain, fatigue) are frequent dose-limiting side effects during IFN treatment of RCC [22]. The frequency and severity of this toxicity are dose dependent. In the author's experience, IFN treatment had to be discontinued or the dose reduced in 57% of the 77 patients receiving IFN 18–36 $\times$ 10^6 U thrice weekly intramuscularly. Creagan et al. [6] combined IFN 20 $\times$ 10^6 U/m^2 given thrice weekly with acetylsalicylic acid in an attempt to reduce subjective toxicity. This combination did not seem to decrease the side effects, but the authors reported a response rate of 34% which was considerably higher than the 15%–20% reported in most other studies using single drug treatment with IFN.

[1] The Norwegian Radium Hospital, Montebello, N-0310 Oslo 3, Norway

F.M.J. Debruyne et al. (Eds.)
Immunotherapy of Renal Cell Carcinoma

Table 1. Interferon plus vinblastine in metastatic renal cell carcinoma: response rates (RR) in phase II studies

Reference		BR[a]
Figlin	(1985)	3/23
Bergerat	(1988)	17/40
Schornagel	(1989)	9/56
Fosså	(1987)	5/28
Cetto	(1987)	8/18
Rizzo	(1989)	5/18
Total		47/183 (25%)

[a] No. of responders/evaluable patients

Table 2. Interferon (IFN) plus vinblastine (VB) in metastatic renal cell carcinoma: results in randomized studies

Reference		IFN	IFN + VB
		Response rates	
Smalley	(1989)	10/82	7/83
Fosså[a]	(1988)	6/86	20/91
Fosså[b]	(1989)	5/24	4/25
		Survival	
Smalley (2 years)	(1989)	7%	7%
Fosså[a] (median)	(1989)	263 days	276 days
Fosså[b] (2 years)	(1990)	30%	35%

[a] European multicenter study
[b] Single institution experience

IFN Combined with Cytostatic Agents

In vitro studies and animal experience have shown a synergistic effect of the combined application of IFN and cytostatic agents [1, 3, 20, 29, 30]. Vinblastine (VB) is claimed to be the most effective cytostatic drug in RCC, with a 25% response rate [17]. It has been combined with IFN in many phase II studies involving RCC (Table 1). In such limited series of highly selected patients, the combination seems to increase the response rate to > 20%. In randomized studies, however, these observations have not been consistently confirmed (Table 2). In addition no survival benefit has been demonstrated for patients who received this combination.

IFN has also been combined with other cytostatic drugs in the treatment of RCC without any definite increase in the response rates (Table 3).

Table 3. Interferon plus cytostatic drugs (other than vinblastine: response rates (RR)

Combination with		RR[a]
Doxorubicin	(Muss et al. 1985)	0/15
Cyclophosphamide	(Walder et al. 1988)	1/25
Cisplatin + 5-fluorouracil + doxorubicin + mitomycin C	(Dexeus et al. 1989)	2/16
Total		3/56

[a] No. of responses/evaluable patients

IFN Combined with Hormonal Agents

In an attempt to reduce the clinical toxicity during IFN treatment the drug was combined with corticosteroids in preliminary studies without an obvious reduction of the response rate [2, 12]. The subjective treatment-related morbidity decreased significantly.

In a subsequent phase II study performed by the author, 5 of 23 patients showed an objective response after receiving IFN 18×10^6 U thrice weekly combined with prednisone 10–20 mg daily orally. There was a marked reduction of subjective side effects when compared with a preceding phase II study using similar IFN doses (Table 4). This combination treatment did not have any impact on the hematological or biochemical toxicity. In a still continuing study the IFN dose was increased to 27×10^6 U thrice weekly, again combined with 10–20 mg prednisone orally daily. So far, 4 of 19 evaluable patients have shown a partial response.

Porzolt et al. [23] combined low doses of IFN with medroxyprogesterone acetate without any obvious increase of the response rate (response rate: 2/46). The combination of IFN plus VB plus tamoxifen did not prove to be more effective than IFN alone [9].

IFN Combined with Other Cytokines

Recently, IFN was combined with other cytokines in the treatment of RCC (IFNγ, tumor necrosis factor, interleukin-2). The clinical experience with these combinations will be discussed in detail in other chapters of this book. From Table 5 it appears that the combination of IFN with interleukin-2 may increase the response rate in RCC, but considerable toxicity has to expected when using high-dose combinations of different cytokines. In conclusion:

1. In today's routine clinical practice, IFN is the drug of choice in patients with metastatic RCC who are candidates for systemic treatment. Doses of 10×10^6 U/m^2 should be given thrice weekly, and treatment should continue for

Table 4. Interferon (IFN) plus prednisone (P) vs IFN alone (historical control group): response rates and clinical toxicity

	IFN + P	IFN
No. of patients	23	27
Response rates[a]	5/23	5/24
Tolerability*		
Very good/good	19	9
Poor	4	18
Flulike symptoms*		
None/mild	21	9
Moderate	2	7
Severe	–	11
Weight loss > 5%	8/22	13/20
Toxicity-related dose reduction/ discontinuation of IFN*	2	11

* $P < 0.01$ (χ^2 test)
[a] No. of responses/evaluable patients

Table 5. Interferon (IFN) plus other cytokines: response rates (RR)

Combination with	Reference	RR[a]
IFNγ	(Quesada et al. 1988)	5/48
IFNγ (low dose)	(Foon et al. 1988)	2/47
IFNγ (high dose)	(Geboers et al. 1988)	6/24
Tumor necrosis factor[b]	(de Mulder et al. 1989)	0/14
Interleukin-2	(Markowitz et al. 1989)	3/14
Interleukin-2[c]	(Krigel et al. 1988)	6/21
Total		22/168

[a] No. of responses/evaluable patients
[b] Combined with IFNγ
[c] Combined with IFNβ

at least 2 months if progression is not observed within this time. A 15%–20% response rate can be expected, especially in patients with lung metastases.

2. The disadvantages of IFN treatment are its subjective morbidity and the relatively high expense of the treatment.
3. There is no reason to combine IFN with VB or other cytostatic drugs except in an adequate trial.
4. The combination with IFN and prednisone seems to decrease the toxicity without obvious reduction of the response rate. This combination should be investigated in future studies.

5. The combination of IFN with other cytokines, especially with interleukin-2, appears to be a step forward in the treatment of metastatic RCC with biological response modifiers.

References

1. Aapro MS, Alberts DS, Salmon SE (1983) Interaction of human leukocyte interferon with vincra alkaloids and other chemotherapeutic agents against human tumors in clonogenic assay. Cancer Chemother Pharmacol 10:161–166
2. Abdi EA (1988) Combination of interferon and prednisone in human cancer. Eur J Clin Oncol 24:723–724
3. Balkwill FR, Moodie EM (1984) Positive interactions between human interferon and cyclophosphamide or adriamycin in a human tumor model system. Cancer Res 44:904–908
4. Bergerat J-P, Herbrecht R, Dufour P, Jocqmin D, Bollack C, Prevot G, Bailly G, de Garis S, Juraschek F, Oberlin F (1988) Combination of recombinant alpha-2A and vinblastine in advanced renal cell cancer. Cancer 62:2320–2324
5. Cetto GL, Franceschi T, Chiarion-Sileni V, Bellini A, Molino AM, Paccagnella A (1987) Recombinant alpha-2 interferon (IFN) and vinblastine (VBL) in metastatic renal cell carcinoma (MRCC): Phase I-II study. Proc Ecco 4, Abstr no 229
6. Creagan ET, Buckner JC, Hahn RG, Richardson RR, Schaid DJ, Kovach JS (1988) An evaluation of recombinant leukocyte A interferon with aspirin in patients with metastatic renal cell cancer. Cancer 61:1787–1791
7. Mulder P de, Debruyne F, Rikken G, Franssen M, van Hoesel Q, Damsma O (1989) Recombinant(r) tumor necrosis factor alpha(NFa-a) and interferon (IFN)-gamma(g) in the treatment of advanced renal cell carcinoma (RCC). Proc Asco 8: Abstract no 560
8. Dexeus FH, Logothetis CJ, Sella A, Finn L (1989) Interferon alternating with chemotherapy for patients with metastatic renal cell carcinoma. Am J Clin Oncol (CCT) 12:350–354
9. Diedrich H, Freund M, Schmoll H-J, Wilke H, v Wussow P (1987) Phase II-trial of a combination therapy with vinblastin (VBL), alpha-human-leukocyte-interferon (HU IFN-alpha) and tamoxifen in advanced renal cell carcinoma (RCC). Proc Ecco 4, Abstract no 229
10. Foon K, Doroshow J, Bonnem E, Fefer A, Graham S, Grosh B et al. (1988) A prospective randomized trial of α-2b-interferon/y-interferon or the combination in advanced metastatic renal cell carcinoma. J Biol Res Mod 7:540–545
11. Figlin RA, De Kernion JB, Maldazys J, Sarna G (1985) Treatment of renal cell carcinoma with alfa (human leucocyte) interferon and vinblastine combination: A phase I-II trial. Cancer Treat Rep 69:263–267
12. Fosså SD (1987) Improved subjective tolerability of interferon by combination with prednisolone. Eur J Cancer Clin Oncol 23:875–876
13. Fosså SD, De Garis ST (1987) Further experience with recombinant interferon alfa-2a with vinblastine in metastatic renal cell carcinoma: A progress report. Int J Cancer 1:35–40
14. Fosså SD, Cavalli F, Otto U, Bauer HW, Oberling JM, Achtnich U et al. (1988) Randomized study of roferon-A (IFN) with or without vinblastine (VBL) in advanced or metastatic renal cell cancer (RCC). Proc ASCO 7, 118: Abstract no 453
15. Fosså SD, Raabe N, Moe B (1989) Recombinant interferon-alpha with or without vinblastine in metastatic renal carcinoma. Results of a randomized phase II study. Br J Urol 64:468–471

16. Geboers ADH, de Mulder PHM, Debruyne FMJ, Strijk SP, Damsma O (1988) Alpha and gamma interferon in treatment of advanced renal cell carcinoma. Sem Surg Oncol 4:191–194
17. Hrusheksy WJ, Murphy GP (1977) Current study of the therapy of advanced renal carcinoma. J Surg Oncol 9:277
18. Krigel R, Padavik K, Rudolph A, Comis R (1988) Phase II study of recombinant interleukin-2 (rIL-2) plus recombinant beta interferon (IFN-β) in advanced renal cell carcinoma. Proc ASCO 7: Abstract no 509
19. Markowitz A, Talpaz M, Lee K, Parkinson D, Doig R, Rothberg J et al. (1989) Phase I-II study of recombinant interleukin-2 (rIL-2) plus recombinant interferon-α2A (rIFN-α) in renal cell carcinoma (RCC). Proc ASCO 8: Abstract no 568
20. Miyoshi T, Ogawa S, Kanamori T, Masahiro N, Namba MY (1983) Interferon potentiates cytotoxic effects of 5-fluorouracil on cell proliferation of established human cell lines originating from neoplastic tissues. Cancer Lett 17:239–247
21. Muss HB, Welander C, Caponera M, Reavis K, Cruz JM, Cooper MR et al. (1985) Interferon and doxorubicin in renal cell carcinoma. Cancer Treat Report 69:721–722
22. Muss HB (1988) The role of biological response modifiers in metatatic renal cell carcinoma. Sem Oncol 15 (Suppl) 5:30–34
23. Porzolt F, Messerer D, Hautmann R, Gottwald A, Sparwasser H, Stockamp K, Aulitzky W et al. (1988) Treatment of advanced renal cell cancer with recombinant interferon alpha as a single agent and in combination with medroxyprogesterone acetate. A randomized multicenter trial. J Cancer Res Clin Oncol 114:95–100
24. Quesada JR, Evans L, Saks SR, Guttermann JU (1988) Recombinant interferon alpha and gamma in combination as treatment for metastatic renal cell carcinoma. J Biol Resp Mod 7:234–239
25. Rizzo M, Bartoletti R, Selli C, Sicignano A, Criscuolo D (1989) Interferon alpha-2a and vinblastine in the treatment of metastatic renal carcinoma. Eur Urol 16:271–277
26. Schornagel HJ, Verweij J, ten Bokkel Huinink WW, Klijn JGM, de Mulder PHM, Debruyne FMJ, van Deijk WA et al. (1989) Phase II study of recombinant interferon alpha-2a and vinblastine in advanced renal cell carcinoma. J Urol 142:253–256
27. Smalley R, Neidhart J, Harris J, Anderson S, Rinehart J, Laszlo J et al. (1989) Pulmonary metastases from renal cell carcinoma. Proc ASCO 8: Abstract no 508
28. Wadler S, Einzig I, Dutcher JP, Ciobano N, Landau L, Wiernik PH (1988) Phase II trial or recombinant alpha-2b-interferon and low-dose cyclophosphamide in advanced melanoma and renal cell carcinoma. Am J Clin Oncol 11:55–59
29. Welander C, Gaines JT, Homesley HD et al. (1983) In vitro synergistic effects of recombinant human interferon alpha$_2$ (rIFN-$_{\alpha 2}$) and doxorubicin on human tumor cell lines. Proc ASCO 2:42
30. Yamamoto S, Tanaka H, Kanamori T et al. (1983) In vitro studies on potentiation of cytotoxic effects of anticancer drugs by interferon on a human neoplastic cell line (HeLa). Cancer Lett 20:131–138

Recombinant Interferon Alpha Plus Vinblastine in Metastatic Renal Cell Cancer: Updated Results

C. Bollack[1], D. Jacqmin[1], J.P. Bergerat[2], J. Ford[2], R. Herbrecht[2], P. Dufour[2], F. Oberling[2], G. Prevost[3], P. Salze[3], and J. Jurascheck[4]

Introduction

Recombinant interferon alpha (IFNα) has been shown to be effective in the treatment of metastatic renal cell cancer (RCC) with response rates in the order of 5%–15% [1–4]. In the hope of improving these results, in 1984 we started a phase I-II study of the combination of IFNα-2a with vinblastine in advanced RCC. Twenty-one patients were entered in this study, in which a dose escalation program permitted us to define the maximal tolerated doses of both drugs in this population. The combination was effective at tolerable doses, and the response rate (39% complete and partial remission, CR + PR) was very encouraging [5]. Based on the results of this first study, we have been conducting since 1985 a phase II study combining fixed doses of IFNα-2a and vinblastine, the preliminary results of which have been published elsewhere [6]. In the present paper we wish to update our experience with this combined therapy in 71 patients with metastatic RCC and to present some information on the prognostic factors, the duration of remission, and the impact on survival.

Methods

Eligibility Criteria

Criteria for inclusion in the study were the presence of metastatic lesions measurable in two dimensions, confirmed progression of these lesions over an observation period of 1 month or longer without treatment, a Karnofsky's index greater than 60%, a serum creatinine of less than 150 μmol/l, and normal serum calcium. Patients with cerebral metastases and those with a history of radiotherapy for indicator lesions or of IFN or vinblastine treatment were not considered eligible.

[1] Service de Chirurgie Urologique, C.H.U. de Strasbourg, 67091 Strasbourg, France
[2] Service d'Onco-Hématologie, C.H.U. de Strasbourg, 67091 Strasbourg, France
[3] Service de Radiothérapie, C.H.R. de Mulhouse, France
[4] Service d'Urologie, C.H.R. de Mulhouse, France

F.M.J. Debruyne et al. (Eds.)
Immunotherapy of Renal Cell Carcinoma

Patients' Characteristics

Between March 1984 and September 1988, 71 patients (58 men and 13 women, median age 60 years, range 27–74 years) with histologically proven metastatic adenocarcinoma were included in the study. In 32 patients metastases were identified at initial diagnosis, and in the remaining 39 the occurrence of metastases was delayed by 1–120 months. Some 69 patients had been treated by nephrectomy (in 6 after preoperative embolization of the renal artery). The other 2 patients were treated by embolization alone. Three patients had been treated previously by chemotherapy, and two had undergone radiotherapy (not directed on indicator lesions).

Treatment

The recombinant IFNα-2a used (Roferon-A, Roche Products) was donated by Hoffmann-La Roche Laboratories (Basle, Switzerland). During the initial phase I-II study involving 21 patients, the treatment began with a dose of 10×10^6 IU/m^2 given by intramuscular injection three times a week, and this dose was increased by 2.5×10^6 IU/m^2 every 2 weeks up to a maximum of 20×10^6 IU/m^2, provided the drug was sufficiently well tolerated. Vinblastine was administered intravenously every 3 weeks starting from the first day of treatment with an initial dose of 0.075 mg/kg; this dose was increased by steps of 0.025 mg/kg every 3 weeks, if it was tolerated up to a maximum of 0.15 mg/kg.

The subsequent group of 50 patients were treated with fixed doses of 18×10^6 IU IFN by intramuscular injection three times a week and 0.10 mg/kg vinblastine given intravenously every 3 weeks starting on the first day of treatment, as determined from the first study.

Patients in whom disease progression was observed at the end of not less than 2 months were withdrawn from the study. In patients with PR or disease stabilisation, the treatment was continued for a period of 1 year. In the event of CR, the treatment was maintained for 6 months and then discontinued.

Results

The results of the program of increasing dosages with the first group have been published elsewhere [5]; none of the patients tolerated the theoretical maximum dose for a prolonged period. The doses were limited due to nonhematologic side effects in 10 patients and hematologic and nonhematologic side effects in 5 patients. The side effects observed in the 50 patients in the second study are summarized in Table 1.

Table 1. Side effects observed in 50 evaluable patients treated with fixed doses of interferon and vinblastine

Flulike syndrome	86%
Severe asthenia	70%
Acute anorexia	30%
Weight loss > 5%	24%
Leucopenia < 3000	24%
Gastrointestinal disorders	22%
Confusion	8%
Dizziness	6%
Increased liver enzymes	4%
Bronchospasm	4%
Peripheral neuropathy	2%
Epilepsy	2%
Thrombocytopenia > 75 000	2%

Response to Therapy

It was possible to evaluate 65 of the 71 patients for a response. The causes of nonevaluability were major protocol violation in one patient and early discontinuation before 6 weeks of therapy without evidence of progressive disease in five. Of these five, one patient underwent surgery on the indicator lesion after 1 month of therapy, one patient was given radiotherapy to the indicator lesion after 5 weeks, one patient refused to continue treatment because of severe asthenia, and treatment was discontinued in two because of side effects (major flulike symptoms and asthenia in one, peripheral neuropathy presumably related to therapy in the other). Two of these six nonevaluable patients died within 1 month from intercurrent complications unrelated to the treatment. From the 65 patients suitable for evaluation we recorded 3 CR, 21 PR, 18 instances of stability (SD), and 23 progressions (PD), giving an overall objective response rate (RR) of 34%. Although the difference was not significant, there was a tendency towards a higher response rate in patients with one or two metastatic sites (RR = 21%). An analysis of response by metastatic site is shown in Table 2. The highest response rate was observed with lung metastases (45%). Approximately 30% of pleural, bone, and liver metastases responded to therapy. Abdominal locoregional recurrences displayed a lower response rate (19%). For other sites the numbers were too small to make an appraisal for the response rate. The response rate was not related to the performance status, though it should be noted that patients with a Karnofsky status of less than 70% were not eligible for this trial.

The three CRs were observed after 3–9 months of treatment in three male patients aged 60, 64, and 68 years; two suffered combined lung and bone metastases, and the third had lung metastases only.

Table 2. Response to treatment arranged by organ with metastasis

Site of metastasis	No. of patients	Complete and partial remissions	Stability and progression of disease
Lung	47	21 (45%)	26 (55%)
Pleura	9	3 (33%)	6 (67%)
Bone	13	4 (31%)	9 (69%)
Liver	7	2 (29%)	7 (71%)
Abdominal recurrence	16	3 (19%)	13 (81%)
Superficial lymph nodes	5	1	4
Skin	3	1	2
Contralateral kidney	2	–	2
Bronchi	1	–	1

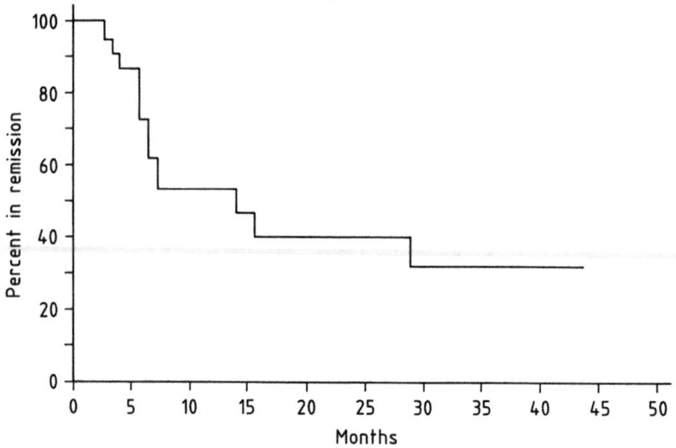

Fig. 1. Survival without relapse in 24 responding patients

Duration of Remission and Survival

Figure 1 shows the predicted duration of remission for the 24 responding patients. The median duration of remission is 13.5 months. Four responding patients are still under therapy. Eleven responding patients relapsed before the completion of 1 year's therapy; nine of these relapsed patients are dead, two are still alive. The median survival of this group of patients who relapsed whilst on-therapy is 13 months. Among the nine patients who completed 1 year of treatment with continuing response, three relapsed 3.5, 5, and 16 months after discontinuation of therapy, while six remain in remission after 25–48 months. The median duration of remission in patients who completed 1 year of therapy is better than 28 months, and the median survival is more than 38 months.

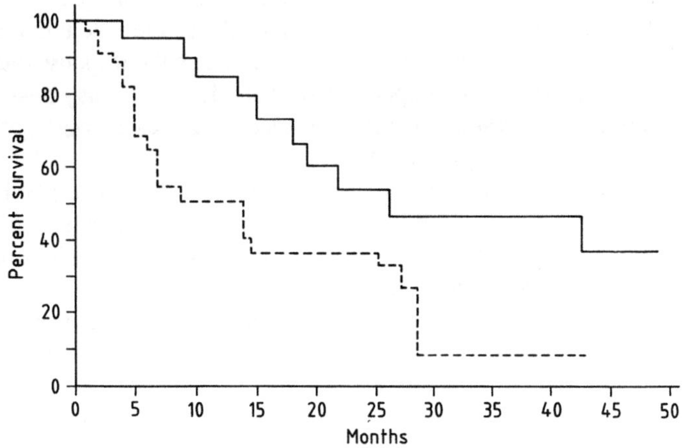

Fig. 2. Survival of responding (n = 24, *upper*) and of nonresponding patients (n = 41, *lower*)

Figure 2 illustrates the survival of responding and nonresponding patients. The median survival of responding patients is 26.5 months, and the predicted 3-year survival rate is 47%. The median survival of nonresponding patients is 12 months, and the predicted 3-year survival rate is below 10%.

Discussion

In our experience, the combinatioin of IFNα and vinblastine is clearly effective in the treatment of metastatic RCC. Its superiority over IFNα alone has now been proven in a multicenter phase III trial [7]. These results suggest the existence of an in vivo synergism between the two drugs. However, other studies of similar combinations in metastatic RCC have given rather irregular results, with response rates ranging from 16% to 36% [7–11]. In an effort to understand the factors which may influence the response and explain the particularly good results which we observed in the present study, the following points should be emphasized:

1. The type of IFN may be of importance. Neidhart and colleagues evaluated the combination of lymphoblastoid IFN and vinblastine. Their conclusion was that the treatment was not tolerable at an effective dose [10].
2. The dose of IFNα is probably of crucial importance. Two randomized trials have shown that low doses are less effective than intermediate or high doses in advanced RCC [12, 13]. A trial evaluating the combination of low doses of IFN and vinblastine concluded that it was more toxic and not more effective than IFN alone [11]. The combination of intermediate doses of IFN and vinblastine as in the present study is often poorly tolerated, especially during the first weeks, and the compliance of the patient and of the treating physician may influence

the response. In this respect we emphasize that no patient in our study received less than 30×10^6 IU/m^2 IFN per week for the whole duration of treatment.

3. The duration of treatment may also influence the response rate. Premature discontinuation of therapy in patients with stable disease may miss potential responders since partial responses were observed as late as 18 weeks after the beginning of treatment in the present study.
4. Among the eligibility criteria, the requirement for a good performance status (> 70%) selects a population of patients who are able to tolerate this treatment and are also more likely to respond than patients who are in a poor general condition. Moreover, the requirement for bidimensionally measurable lesions left out some patients with nonmeasurable bone metastases.
5. Finally, considering the characteristics of the patients entered in the present study, two more factors may have contributed to the particularly high response rate observed. Firstly, the percentage of lung metastases was high (70%) with 30% of the patients presenting with lung metastases alone; it has been established that the lung is the site most likely to respond to IFN therapy in metastatic RCC. Secondly, it has been shown that IFNα is more effective in nephrectomized than in nonnephrectomized patients [14]. In the present study, although nephrectomy was not a mandatory eligibility criteria, most patients (61 of 63) had been previously nephrectomized, even when metastatic at the time of diagnosis.

Taken together, these observations suggest that RCC patients most likely to respond to the IFNα-vinblastine combination therapy are those who have been previously nephrectomized and present with a good performance status, a low number of metastatic sites, and metastases in the lung rather than at other sites. The analysis of remission and survival data shows that the prognosis of responding patients who relapse early (while on therapy) is as poor as that of nonresponding patients. Only patients who remain in PR or CR after completion of 1 year of therapy experience prolonged remission (median > 28 months) and survival (median > 38 months). The proportion of CRs is low, and it is unfortunately likely that none of these patients has been cured by the treatment. However, there is a survival benefit as the median survival and the 3-year rate of the whole population entered in this study are 20 months and 28%, respectively, while those of historical controls not treated by interferon are less than 10 months and less than 10%, respectively.

Such observations of very long remissions and the occurrence of PRs reaching sponteously CRs after the end of treatment have also been reported with lymphokine-activated killer cell and interleukin-2 treatment, and suggest that such therapies modify the host-tumor relationships in the long-term. Although modest, these results represent considerable progress in comparison with those of previously available therapies and justify continuing the investigation of biological response modifiers in this disease and evaluating new therapeutic strategies and combinations with such agents.

References

1. Kempf RA, Grunberg SM, Daniels JR et al. (1983) Recombinant interferon alpha 2 in a phase II study of renal cell carcinoma. Proc Am Soc Clin Oncol 3:59
2. Krown SE, Eizing AI, Abrahamson JD, Oettgen HF (1983) Treatment of advanced renal cell cancer with recombinant leucocyte A interferon. Proc Am Soc Clin Oncol 2:58
3. Neidhardt JA (1986) Interferon therapy for the treatment of renal cancer. Cancer 57:1696–1699
4. Quesada JE, Swanson DA, Trindale A, Guttermann JV (1983) Renal cell carcinoma: Antitumor effects of leucocyte interferon. Cancer Res 43:940–943
5. Bergerat JP, Dufour P, Soyer Y et al. (1987) Traitement des adénocarcinomes rénaux métastatiques par l'association interféron recombinant alpha-2a et vinblastine. Presse Med 16:1953–1956
6. Bergerat JP, Herbrecht R, Dufour P et al. (1988) Combination of recombinant interferon alpha 2a and vinblastine in advanced renal cell cancer. Cancer 62:2320–2324
7. Fossa SD, Cavalli F, Otto U et al. (1988) Randomized study of Roferon-A with or without vinblastine in advanced or metastatic renal cell cancer. Proc Am Soc Clin Oncol 7:118
8. Fossa SD, de Garis ST, Heier MS et al. (1986) Recombinant interferon alpha-2a with or without vinblastine in metastatic renal cell carcinoma. Cancer 57:1700–1704
9. Schornagel J, Verwey J, ten Bokkel Huinink W et al. (1987) Phase II study of recombinant interferon alpha-2 (IFN) and vinblastine (V) in advanced renal carcinoma (ARC). Proc Am Soc Clin Oncol 6:106
10. Neidhart J, Harris J, Tuttle R (1987) A randomized study of wellferon (WFN) with or without vinblastine (VLB) in advanced renal cancer. Proc Am Soc Clin Oncol 6:239
11. Figlin RA, de Kernion JB, Maldazys J, Sarna G (1985) Treatment of renal cell carcinoma with alfa (human leucocyte) interferon and vinblastine combination: A phase I-II trial. Cancer Treat Rep 69:263–267
12. Kirkwood JM, Harris JE, Very R et al. (1985) Randomized study of low and high doses of leucocyte alfa-interferon in metastatic renal cell carcinoma. Am Cancer Soc Collaborative Trial Cancer Res 45:863–871
13. Quesada JR, Guttermann JV, Rios A (1983) Investigational therapy of renal cell carcinoma with recombinant alfa-interferon. Prof Am Assoc Cancer Res 24–195
14. Vugrin D, Hood L, Lazlo J (1985) A phase II trial of high-dose human lymphoblastoid alpha interferon in patients with advanced renal carcinoma. Cancer Treat Rep 69:817

Monotherapy and Combination Therapy with Interferon-α, Interferon-γ, and Tumor Necrosis Factor-α in Metastatic Renal Cell Carcinoma

P.H.M de Mulder[1], M.P.H. Franssen[2], C.J.A. Punt[1], and F.M.J. Debruyne[2]

Introduction

Patients with renal cell carcinoma (RCC) currently have few therapeutic options once the disease has become metastatic. Approximately 25% of patients have metastatic disease at the time of first presentation [34]. The median survival for those patients is 6–12 months [6]. Spontaneous regression of metastases after tumor nephrectomy is less than 1% [24]. Hormonal treatment results in a small proportion (0%–10%) of objective responses, which are often incomplete and of short duration [14]. Single-agent chemotherapy adds little in terms of tumor response. Combination chemotherapy induces a slightly higher response rate, but no clearly definable improvement in survival has been demonstrated [14, 38]. In view of the unusual natural history of the tumor, such as the abovementioned spontaneous regressions and the dormant tendency of metastases, especially pulmonary metastases, an interaction between the host and the tumor has been suggested. For this reason several forms of immunotherapy have been employed, resulting in a limited number of sometimes long-lasting responses [23]. Most emphasis has been given to those forms of immunotherapy which induce stimulation of the immune-effector systems of the host. These approaches are currently described as treatment with biological response modifiers (BRM). Interferons (IFN) are the most extensively tested BRM in metastatic RCC. In this review the achievements with IFN-α, -β and -γ as monotherapy and in combinations will be discussed, and some data will be presented regarding the combination of IFN-γ with tumor necrosis factor-α (TNF-α).

Interferons

The IFN are a group of naturally occurring proteins with potent antiviral, antiproliferative and immunomodulatory properties such as the activation of natural killer cells and macrophages, the increased expression of tumor-associated antigens and the modulation of MHC class I and II antigens. On the basis of their antigenic specificities, a division is made into three main groups. The IFN-α are a group

[1,2] Division of Medical Oncology, Department of Medicine[1] and Department of Urology[2], University Hospital Nijmegen, P.O. Box 9101, 6500 HB, Nijmegen, The Netherlands

F.M.J. Debruyne et al. (Eds.)
Immunotherapy of Renal Cell Carcinoma

of closely related proteins with approximately 75% homology in their amino acid sequences which are produced by macrophages and lymphocytres upon exposure to virus particles and compete with IFN-β for the same receptor. IFN-β is produced by fibroblasts, and IFN-γ is the product of a single gene and is produced by activated T-lymphocytes and natural killer cells [37].

IFN-α is most extensively used in the treatment of advanced RCC, both in the natural and in the recombinant (r) form.

IFN-α

Since the first report that a partially purified human IFN-α preparation could induce the regression of metastatic RCC [30], numerous therapeutic trials have been conducted to assess the efficacy of various IFN-α preparations. The most frequently used IFN are: human leukocyte IFN, lymphoblastoid IFN (αN1), rIFN-α2a, rIFN-α2b and rIFN-α2c. Most studies have provided evidence for modest but reproducible antitumor activity in advanced RCC. From several recently published overviews it is possible to define the place of IFN-α in the treatment of metastatic RCC [3, 13, 15, 18, 25, 35].

Although a randomized study comparing different dose levels, with a sufficient number of patients, has never been performed, IFN-α therapy with an intermediate dose (3–10 $\times$ 10^6 U/day) appears to be more effective than therapy with a low dose (< 3 $\times$ 10^6 U/day) or a high dose (> 10 $\times$ 10^6 U/day). Our own observations with an escalating dose of rIFN-α2c in combination with a fixed dose of rIFN-γ two times weekly s.c. also indicate the existence of a dose-response relationship [12]. In four of seven patients with stable disease (SD) and one of five with progressive disease (PD) being treated with low-dose rIFN-α (2 $\times$ 10^6 IU/m^2 s.c. twice per week), a response was seen after escalation to a median dose of 10 $\times$ 10^6 IU/m^2.

So far, no scheme of administration – cyclic, continuous, five times or three times weekly – has been identified as definitely superior, and no difference has been established between routes – subcutaneous or intramuscular. Intravenous administration is more complicated and may be less effective [15]. The purity of the various IFN-α preparations is not considered critical in view of the very comparable respones found with the natural leukocyte and the three most frequently used recombinant forms [3, 15, 18, 25, 35]. The response rates recorded from adequate trials (those with more than 20 eligible patients and a dose of IFN-α exceeding 3 $\times$ 10^6 U/day, n = 431) vary from 5% to 26% (mean 17%; CR 2% and PR 15%). It is well recognized that the primary tumor and metastases in bone and central nervous system rarely respond to this type of treatment. Furthermore, large tumor masses are less likely to regress than is limited disease [30]. Lung metastases are especially susceptible to IFN treatment [3, 15, 18, 22, 25, 30, 35, 36]. The median survival for responders and nonresponders together is most often less than 1 year.

It is important to realize that patients with a high performance status, lung metastases only and a disease-free period of more than 1 year after tumor nephrectomy have much longer median survival (155 weeks vs 49 weeks for the whole group studied [35]). IFN-α is probably not able to cure patients with RCC, but can induce a meaningful remission in a subgroup of patients. The duration of treatment is uncertain. In an analysis of 288 responders, the response was seen in 76% within 3 months of the commencement of treatment, in 12% between 3 and 6 months and in 12% after more than 6 months of treatment [20]. Patients are rarely treated for longer than 1 year. The side effects of IFN are well known and will not be discussed in detail. However, they constitute a major reason for discontinuation of treatment. The observation of Fossa (presented elsewhere in this monograph) that IFN-α can be combined with corticosteroids without compromising efficacy, and the fact that this is also true for nonsteroidal antiinflammatory drugs [4], point to effective ways of diminishing side effects.

IFN-β

The experience with IFN-β is still very limited, and it is therefore too early to draw any conclusions. It has been hypothesized that IFN-β-serine, a mutein recombinant IFN that is tolerated at a dose five- to tenfold higher than IFN-α, might induce a higher response rate. However, in a recently published phase II study the response rate was 4/25 patients (one CR) [17], which is the same as could be expected from IFN-α.

Table 1. Studies on the efficacy of rIFN-γ in advanced renal cell carcinoma

Reference	Regimen	Route	Dose (mg/m^2)		CR	PR	Response rate (%)
21	7 days/14 days[a]	i.v.	0.3–3	(B)	1/41	3/41	10
22	2/week	i.v.	30–75[c]	(B)	0/13	0/13	0
23	daily[a]	i.v.	0.01–0.05	(G)	0/18	1/18	6
23	daily[a]	i.m.	0.25–1	(G)	0/15	1/15	7
24	3/week[b]	i.v.	0.1	(B)	1/16	4/16	31
25	3/week	i.v.	0.1	(G)	0/32	1/32	3
27	1/week	s.c.	0.1–0.5	(G)	2/16	4/16	30

[a] (*B*), Biogen; (*G*), Genentech Increasing dose
[b] In case of no response after 12 weeks, dosage was increased to 0.5 mg/m^2 five times a week
[c] $\times 10^6$ U/m^2

IFN-γ

The experience with rIFN-γ in RCC is also limited (Table 1). In a phase I-II study with an escalating dose of rIFN-γ (Biogen) i.v. over 7 days every other week, dose-limiting toxicity was observed between 1000 and 3000 $\mu g/m^2$. Tumor responses were already seen at the 300 $\mu g/m^2$ dose level. In 41 patients evaluable for response, one CR and three PR (10%) occurred [11]. In six other patients site-specific responses were seen in lung, lymph node, pleura and liver. No regression of the primary tumor was found in this series, which is comparable with the observations with IFN-α. Using the same IFN with a different schedule (4 h i.v. twice per week) no responses were documented in 13 patients treated in a phase I/II study [33]. The phase II study conducted by Quesada et al. with partially purified IFN-γ was also negative [31]. A remarkable finding was the response rate of 31% (5/16) with IF-γ (Biogen) given as a 4-h infusion three times weekly every other week (100–500 $\mu g/m^2$) [27]. In a study testing the same regimen with IFN-γ (Genentech) only one PR was seen in 32 evaluable patients [2]. Little information is available about the optimal dose, schedule and route of IFN-γ administration. Modification of the host response is frequently restricted to a narrow dose range, and in a recent study optimal modulation by rIFN-γ has been found in the low dose range (100 $\mu g/m^2$) [21]. Against this background the findings of Aulitzky et al. [1] are interesting: they observed a 30% response rate (two CR, four PR) in 16 patients treated with 100 μg IFN-γ (Genentech) s.c. once a week. At this dose a nearly maximum response of serum β_2-microglobulin (nonpolymorphic chain of MHC class I) and neopterin, which represents a functional activation of the monocyte-macrophage system, was found, indicating adequate immune modulation. Patients with refractory disease had significantly lower IFN-γ induced increments of serum β_2-microglobulin than those who achieved a clinical remission or stable disease. A similar pattern was seen for neopterin, but these differences were not statistically significant.

Combination of IFN-α and IFN-γ

On the basis of in vitro observations indicating a synergism between rIFN-γ and rIFN-α [5, 16], combined studies have been initiated. In a phase I study the dose recommended for phase II studies was 0.5×10^6 U/m²/day i.m. of each IFN type, with the possibility of dose escalation if the tolerability was acceptable [19]. The results published so far are disappointing. In three phase II studies [32], 53 patients were treated with a combination of rIFN-α2a and rIFN-γ (Genentech). Thirteen were simultaneously treated with daily i.m. injections of 2×10^6 U/m² rIFN-α2a and rIFN-γ (rIFN-α:rIFN-γ = 1:10 by protein weight). No response was seen in 10 evaluable patients. In the second study, rIFN-α2a and rIFN-γ were also given daily i.m. on a 1:1 protein basis, with the possibility of dose increase. In four of 25 patients a PR was seen, and the regimen was well tolerated, allowing a 25%–50% increment of dose in 75% of the patients. In the third study, an alternating regimen was used: rIFN-γ at 5×10^6 U/m^2 i.m. for 7 days followed by rIFN-α2a at 10×10^6 U/m^2. In 15 evaluable patients, one PR was observed. In a prospective randomized trial, the efficacy of (1) rIFN-α2b in an dose of 2×10^6 U/m^2 i.m. three times a week, (2) rIFN-γ 1×10^6 U/m^2 three times a week and (3) the same doses in combination were tested [10]. The response rates were not different (1/21, 1/21 and 2/47 respectively).

Our Own Observations. In view of the data discussed we studied the efficacy of the combination of an escalating dose of rIFN-α (6 μg/m^2 = 2×10^6 U/m^2 starting dose) and a fixed low dose of rIFN-γ (100 μg/m^2 = 2×10^6 U/m^2) two times weekly s.c. in patients with advanced progressive RCC [12, 29]. After 8 weeks of treatment the dose of rIFN-α was escalated in steps of 6 μg/m^2 until the maximum tolerated dose (MTD) was reached. Thirty-two patients were included: 21 males and 11 females with a mean age of 57.2 years (range 35–72 years). Twenty-nine of them had undergone nephrectomy prior to the start of treatment, the median Karnofsky performance status was 90% (70%–100%), and the disease was predominantly at visceral sites. Thirty-one patients were evaluable for response (one patient was excluded after reaching a CR because retrospectively the first signs of tumor regression were seen before the start of treatment despite earlier well-documented progression 2 months after nephrectomy). Two patients discontinued treatment within 8 weeks due to toxicity, but were included in the response analysis. The overall response rate was 26% (two CR, six PR). Five patients achieved stabilization of disease, and in 16 progressive disease was found. The median response duration for PR was 14 months (range 8–16 months). Both CR patients are off treatment (treatment continued for 1 year after CR was first observed); the response persists in one (23+ months after reaching CR), and the other had a relapse after 22 months. The median time to response was 24 weeks (range 12–36 weeks). The MTD for rIFN-α was 30 μg/m^2 (range 6–36 μg/m^2). Side effects included those known to be associated with IFN treatment. One patient developed septicemia during WHO grade IV leukopenia, from which he recovered fully after discontinuation of IFN. In a subsequent study, 25 patients were treated with a starting dose of 24 μg/m^2 rIFN-α with, if possible, one escalation step of 6 μg/m^2, and the same dose of rIFN-γ (100 μg/m^2). The patient characteristics of this group were comparable with those of the first group. Twenty-three patients were evaluable for response. The overall response rate of this second group was 22% (four CR, one PR, four SD, 12 PD). The median time to response was 12 weeks (range 4–12 weeks), compared with 24 weeks in the first group (range 12–36 weeks). Thus it appears that the higher starting dose of rIFN-α induces a more rapid response. The 11% CR rate for the two studies is a remarkable finding and may indicate a positive effect of rIFN-γ when combined with an optimal dose of rIFN-α [7]. A randomized study to answer this question more definitely is currently being performed by the EORTC genitourinary cooperative group.

Comparing our results with those reported above, the difference in response rate may be explained by our optimal dose of rIFN-γ and by the relatively low dose of rIFN-α used in most other studies (Table 2).

Table 2. Doses of rIFN-α and rIFN-γ and response

rIFN-α (MU/m^2 week)	rIFN-γ (MU/m^2 week)	CR	PR	Response rate (%)	Reference
14	14	0/10	0/10	0	[30]
14	1.4	0/25	4/25	16	[30]
70[a]	35[a]	0/13	1/13	8	[30]
6	3	0/47	2/47	4	[31]
4	4	0/14	0/14	0	[32]
20	4	2/31	6/31	26	[33]

[a] In alternate weeks

In an attempt to monitor the immunomodulatory properties of IFN, we tested the skin reactivity to a standard panel of recall antigens prior to and during treatment and followed neopterin excretion as an indicator of macrophage activation. No persistent changes in response to recall antigens (applied in a standard manner) were observed during IFN treatment, nor was there any difference between responders and nonresponders. Neopterin, measured in the urine after collection and storage under standard conditions, had a pretreatment concentration of 254 ± 174 (mean $\pm$ SD) μmol/mol creatinine in responders and $265 \pm 111 \mu$mol/mol in nonresponders. During treatment, urinary neopterin increased significantly in all cases ($p < 0.01$): to $1125 \pm 713 \mu$mol/mol in responders and $752 \pm 402 \mu$mol/mol in nonresponders. The posttreatment difference between responders and nonresponders was not statistically significant ($p > 0.05$).

Tumor Necrosis Factor

rTNF-α is synthesized and secreted by macrophages and induces hemorrhagic necrosis in murine tumors [26]. Cytotoxic activity has been demonstrated in vitro against various murine and human cell lines. Furthermore, synergistic cytotoxic activity with IFN has been observed. Published observations of the effect of TNF in RCC are scarce. In one phase II study the efficacy and side effects of rTNF-α 50 μg/m^2 i.m. and rIFN-γ 100 μg/m^2 s.c. three times a week in advanced, progressive RCC were investigated [8]. Twenty-one patients were entered, 13 males and 8 females, mean age 54.2 years (range 43–70 years). Patient characteristics were similar to those in the earlier mentioned studies. Seven patients were taken off study due to toxicity: one had bronchospasm, one had thrombosis, four displayed high fever, severe weight loss and nausea and vomiting, and in one patient hemiplegia occurred after one injection due to hemorrhage in a previously not recognized CNS metastasis. One CR and no PR have been found in 14 patients evaluable for response. Three patients had a minor response and 10 had PD. Side effects included high fever, rigors, influenza-like symptoms and anorexia in all patients. In three patients hypercalcemia without signs of progressive disease was a reason for early discontinuation. No significant hematological toxicity was seen. These preliminary data show no activity and considerable toxicity for the combination of rTNF-α and IFN-γ in advanced RCC.

In another study 25 patients (14 with RCC and 11 with malignant melanoma) were treated with an escalating dose of rTNF-α (25–75 $\mu g/m^2$/day); no objective responses were noted [9]. Otto et al. [28] evaluated in a phase I/II trial the toxicity and efficacy of rTNF-α as monotherapy and in combination with rIFN-α2a. Twelve patients received rTNF-α i.v. five times weekly in a dose of 200–300 $\mu g/m^2$, five of them in combination with 12 × 10^6 U rIFN-α2a i.m. three times a week. No responses were seen, and toxicity included fever, chills, influenza-like symptoms, nausea, vomiting, malaise, anorexia and hepato- and myelotoxicity. In a subsequent phase II study rTNF-α was given at a dose of 160 $\mu g/m^2$ i.v. five times a week every 3rd week and rIFN-α2a 18 × 10^6 U i.m. three times a week every week. The preliminary results in seven evaluable patients were one CR, four PR, and one SD. More information is needed to judge the value of this combination in the treatment of advanced RCC.

Conclusion

IFN-α is the most extensively tested IFN in RCC, and the objective response rate (judged on WHO criteria) ranges from 1% to 26%. Pooling of the data gives a response rate of approximately 17%. An intermediate dose is considered optimal. Patients with extensive disease, poor performance status, or bone and central nervous system metastases are unlikely to respond to IFN treatment. Furthermore, regression of the primary tumor, which often constitutes an important tumor mass, rarely occurs. The results with IFN-γ are disappointing in most studies, with a response rate of 0%–10%. Only a limited number of studies have been performed with an optimal dose of rIFN-γ, the positive results in a small group of patients reported by Aulitzky et al. [27] should be confirmed. The results of IFN-α and IFN-γ combination therapy do not seem to be superior to those of IFN-α monotherapy, a randomized study is still ongoing. The available data on TNF in RCC are limited and show no major efficacy, either alone or in combination. The toxicity is considerable. After initial positive experience, the combined treatment with rTNF-α and rIFN-α2a is being investigated further, and we should await the results [28]. Interesting new options currently being tested are combinations of IFN with other cytokines such as IL-2 with and without activated killer cells.

References

1. Aulitzky W, Gastl WE, Aulitzky WE et al. (1989) Successful treatment of metastatic renal cell carcinoma with a biologically active dose of recombinant interferon-gamma. J Clin Oncol 7:1815–1884
2. Bruntsch U, De Mulder PHM, ten Bokkel Huinink WW et al. (1990) Phase II study of recombinant human interferon-gamma in metastatic renal cell carcinoma. J Biol Response Mod 9:335–338
3. Buzaid AC, Todd MB (1989) Therapeutic options in renal cell carcinoma. Semin Oncol 16:12–19
4. Creagan ET, Buckner JC, Hahn RG et al. (1988) An evaluation of recombinant leukocyte A interferon with asperin in patients with metastatic renal cell cancer. Cancer 61:1787–1791
5. Czarniecki CW, Fennie CW, Powers DB et al. (1984) Synergistic antiviral and antiproliferative activities of E. coli derived human alpha, beta, and gamma interferon. J Virol 49:490–496
6. De Forges A, Rey A, Klink M et al. (1988) Prognostic factors in adult metastatic renal carcinoma: A multivariate analysis. Semin Surg Oncol 4:149–154
7. De Mulder PHM, Geboers ADH, Debruyne FMJ et al. (1988) Recombinant interferon alpha and gamma in the treatment of advanced renal cell carcinoma. J Urol 139:294
8. De Mulder PHM, Debruyne F, Rikken G et al. (1989) Recombinant tumor necrosis factor alpha and interferon gamma in the treatment of advanced renal cell carcinoma. Proc Am Soc Clin Oncol 8:A560
9. Figlin R, Dekernion J, Sarna G et al. (1988) Phase II study of recombinant tumor necrosis factor in patients with metastatic renal carcinoma and malignant melanoma. Proc Am Soc Clin Oncol 7:A652
10. Foon K, Doroshow J, Bonnem E et al. (1988) A prospective randomized trial of α2b-interferon/g-interferon or the combination in advanced metastatic renal cell carcinoma. J Biol Response Mod 7:540–545
11. Garnick MB, Reich SD, Maxwell B et al. (1988) Phase I/II study of recombinant interferon gamma in advanced renal cell carcinoma. J Urol 139:251–255
12. Geboers ADH, De Mulder PHM, Debruyne FMJ et al. (1988) Alpha and gamma interferon in the treatment of advanced renal cell carcinoma. Semin Surg Oncol 4:191–194
13. Goldstein D, Laslo J (1986) Interferon therapy in cancer: From imaginon to interferon. Cancer Res 46:4315–4329
14. Harris DT (1983) Hormonal therapy and chemotherapy of renal cell carcinoma. Semin Oncol 10:422–430
15. Horoszewicz JS, Murphy GP (1989) An assessment of the current use of human interferons in therapy of urological cancers. J Urol 142:1173–1180
16. Hubbell HR, Craft JA, Leibowitz P et al. (1987) Synergistic antiproliferative effect of recombinant alpha-interferons with recombinant gamma-interferons. J BNiol Resp Mod 6:141–153
17. Kinney P, Triozzi P, Young D et al. (1990) Phase II trial of interferon-beta-serine in metastatic renal cell carcinoma. J Clin Oncol 8:881–885
18. Krown SE (1987) Interferon treatment of renal cell carcinoma. Current status and future prospects. Cancer 59:647–651
19. Kurzrock R, Rosenblum MG, Quesada JR et al. (1986) Phase I study of a recombinant interferon-alpha and recombinant-gamma in cancert patients. J Clin Oncol 4:1677–1683
20. Levens W, Rubben H, Ingenhag W (1989) Long-term interferon treatment in metastatic renal cell carcinoma. Eur Urol 16:378–381

21. Maluish AE, Urba WJ, Longo DL et al. (1988) The determination of an immunologically active dose of interferon gamma in patients with melanoma. J Clin Oncol 6:434–445
22. Marumo K, Murai M, Hayakawa M et al. (1984) Human lymphoblastoid interferon for advanced renal cell carcinoma. Urology 6:567–571
23. McCune CS (1983) Immunologic therapies in kidney carcinoma. Semin Oncol 10:431–436
24. Montie JE, Stewart BH, Straffon RA et al. (1977) The role of adjunctive nephrectomy in patients with metastatic renal cell carcinoma. J Urol 117:272–275
25. Muss HB (1988) Interferon therapy of metastatic renal cell cancer. Semin Surg Oncol 4:199–203
26. Old LJ (1985) Tumor necrosis factor (TNF). Science 230:630–632
27. Otto U, Conrad S, Schneider AW, Klosterhalfen H (1988) Recombinant interferon gamma in the treatment of metastatic renal cell carcinoma. Arzneim Forsch/Drug Res 38:1658
28. Otto U, Schneider AW, Conrad S et al. (1989) Effektivität und Toxizität von TNF in Kombination mit Alpha 2 Interferon bei Patientenm mit einem metastasierenden Nierenkarzinom. Urologe [A] 28 (Suppl):A3
29. De Mulder PHM, Debruyne FMJ, Franssen MPH et al. (1990) Phase I/II Study of Recombinant Interferon Alpha and Gamma in Advanced Progressive Renal Cell Carcinoma. Cancer Immunol Immunother 31:321–324
30. Quesada JR, Swanson DA, Trindae A et al. (1986) Renal cell carcinoma: Antitumor effects of leucocyte interferon. Cancer Res 46:940–943
31. Quesada JR, Kurzrock R, Sherwin SA et al. (1987) Phase II studies of recombinant human interferon gamma in metastatic renal cell carcinoma. J Biol Response Mod 6:20–27
32. Quesada JR, Evans L, Saks SR et al. (1988) Recombinant interferon alpha and gamma in combination as treatment for metastatic renal cell carcinoma. J Biol Resp Mod 7:234–239
33. Rinehart JJ, Malspeis L, Young D et al. (1986) Phase I/II trial of human recombinant interferon gamma in renal cell carcinoma. J Biol Response Mod 5:300–308
34. Ritchie AWS, Chrisholm GD (1983) The natural history of renal cell carcinoma. Semin Oncol 10:390–400
35. Sarna G, Figlin R, deKernion J (1987) Interferon in renal cell carcinoma. The UCLA experience. Cancer 59:610–612
36. Vugrin D, Hood L, Taylor W et al. (1985) Phase II study of human lymphoblastoid interferon in patients with advanced renal carcinoma. Cancer Tr Rep 69:817–820
37. Wagstaff J, Melief KJ (1987) Lymphokines and cytokines. In: Pinedo HM, Longo DL, Chabner BA (eds) Cancer chemotherapy and biological response modifiers, Annual 9. Elsevier, Amsterdam, p 432
38. Yagoda A, Bander NH (1989) Failure of cytotoxic chemotherapy, 1983–1988, and the emerging role of monoclonal antibodies for renal cancer. Urol Int 44:338–345

Treatment of Advanced Renal Cell Carcinoma by Systemic Low-Dose Recombinant Interleukin-2

Y. Aso[1], H. Tazaki[2], T. Umeda[1], K. Marumo[2], and Recombinant Human Interleukin-2 (S-6820) Research Group on Renal Cell Carcinoma (Chairman: Fumimaro Takaku)[3]

Introduction

In 1976, Morgan and his associates [1] first reported that interleukin-2 (IL-2) was a T-cell growth factor. Since then, various biological activities of IL-2 [2] have been elucidated, including proliferation of T cells, natural killer (NK) cells, and lymphokine-activated killer (LAK) cells; induction of cytotoxicity of killer T cells, NK cells, LAK cells, and monocytes; induction of lymphokine production such as interferon, IL-3, -4, -5, -6, colony stimulating factor, and tumor necrosis factor; and induction of receptors.

Since Rosenberg and his associates [3] reported the clinical efficacy of the combination of adoptive immunotherapy and IL-2 on renal cell carcinoma, melanoma, and colonic cancer, the usefulness of IL-2 for malignancy has been investigated at various institutes [4, 5]. We, the Japanese urological group consisting of 27 institutes, have studied the effectiveness of a low-dose IL-2 treatment for 89 patients with advanced renal cell carcinoma from October 1985 until December 1988. This presentation reports the results of our study.

[1] Department of Urology, Faculty of Medicine, The University of Tokyo, 7-3-1 Hongo, Bunkyo-ku, Tokyo 113, Japan

[2] Department of Urology, Keio University Medical School, Shinano-machi, Tokyo 160, Japan

[3] Recombinant Human Interleukin 2 (S 6820) Research Group on Renal Cell Carcinoma. Departments of Urology: The University of Tokyo (Yoshio Aso, Takashi Umeda), Keio University (Hiroshi Tazaki, Ken Marumo), Hokkaido University (Tomohiko Koyanagi), Sapporo Medical College (Yoshiaki Kumamoto, Taikji Tsukamoto), Iwate Medical University (Tsutomu Ohori), Tohoku University (Seiichi Orikasa), Jichi Medical School (Yasuyuki Yonese), The University of Tsukuba (Kenkichi Koiso), Nihon University (Takashi Kishimoto, Kiyoki Okada), Juntendo University (Ryuichi Kitagawa), Nippon Medical School (Masao Akimoto), The Jikei University (Toyohei Machida), National Cancer Center (Tadao Kakizoe), Tokai University (Nobuo Kawamura), Yokosuka Kyosai Hospital (Yoshiaki Satomi), Toyama Medical and Pharaceutical University (Takashi Katayama), Kanazawa University (Haruo Hisazumi), Japanese Red Cross Nagoya Second Hospital (Koji Obata), Hamamatsu University (Kazuki Kawabe), Mie University (Juichi Kawamura), Kyoto University (Osamu Yoshida, Yasunori Nishio), Osaka City University (Masanobu Maekawa), Okayama University (Hiroyuki Ohmori), Kyushu University (Joichi Kumazawa, Toyofumi Ueda), University of the Ryukyus (Akira Osawa)

F.M.J. Debruyne et al. (Eds.)
Immunotherapy of Renal Cell Carcinoma

Table 1. Background of the patients in the present study

Characteristic	*n*	Characteristic	*n*
Eligible cases	65	Prior therapy:	
Males/females	49/16	Nephrectomy	55
Age (years):		Chemotherapy	21
< 50	6	Immunotherapy	27
50 59	23	Radiation	4
60 69	22	Maximum daily dose:	
70 79	13	0.5×10^6 U body	4
≥ 80	1	1.0×10^6 U body	44
Performance status:		$\geq 2.0 \times 10^6$ U body	17
0	21	Treatment duration (weeks):	
1	29	4– 8	30
2	8	8–12	17
3	4	12–16	5
4	3	16–52	10
Histological type:		≥52	3
Common type	49		
Clear cell subtype	31		
Granular cell subtype	3		
Mixed subtype	15		
Pleomorphic type	1		
Unknown	15		

Methods and Materials

IL-2 (1×10^6 units per body) was given by 2-hours intravenous drip infusion every day for more than 28 days. If tolerated, the dose was escalated up to 3×10^6 units per patient daily. For three outpatients, it was also administered subcutaneously.

Eligibility for the study included a 4 weeks' treatment-free period after any previous therapy except for antimetabolites and biological response modifiers (10–14 days) and a 7-days interval after nephrectomy. Although performance status 4 (PS-4) patients were excluded, those with immobilization due to brain or bone metastases were eligible for the study.

Among 89 entries, 12 patients were not eligible for the study because of lack of a drug-free interval (8), absence of evaluable lesions (2), double cancer (1), and PS-4 (1). Reasons for dropping out included 6 interruptions with the treatment duration shorter than 28 days due to adverse effects, 2 deaths during the treatment, 2 administrations of other drugs, and 2 not evaluable lesions leading to lack of comparable estimation before and after treatment. Excluding these 24, 65 patients were evaluated in the study. Their backgrounds are shown in Table 1, including sex ratio, age distribution, PS, histological classification, prior therapy, maximum daily dose, and treatment duration. Of the 65, 59 received prior treatments including nephrectomy (55). The dose of 10^6 units per body was most frequently given. In

Table 2. Efficacy of recombinant interleukin-2 on renal cell carcinoma

	n	Percentage
Complete response	3	4.6
Partial response	7	10.8
Minor response	1	1.5
Stabel disease	26	40.0
Progressive disease	28	43.1
Total	65	100.0

Table 3. Background of responders and nonresponders to recombinant interleukin-2

	Age	Sex		Performance status				
	Mean ± SD	M	F	0	1	2	3	4
Total (65 patients)	61 ± 10	49	16	21	29	8	4	3
Responders (10 : 3CR + 7PR)	59 ± 9	8	2	3	6	1		
Nonresponders 55 : 1MR + 26SD + 28PD)	61 ± 10	41	14	18	23	7	4	3

75 patients (excluding 2 with simultaneous use of other drugs of the 77 eligible cases), side effects were evaluated.

Results

The response of the 65 evaluable patients is shown in Table 2. The numbers of complete, partial, and minor response (CR, PR, MR), stable disease (SD) and progression (PD) were 3 (4.6%), 7 (10.8%), 1 (1.5%), 26 (40.0%), and 28 (43.1%), respectively. The response rate including CR and PR was 15.4% (10/65). Responders are mostly patients with a low PS – usually 0 or 1 (9/10). There was only 1 responder among patients with a PS of 2 or more (Table 3).

Response of individual metastatic organs was analyzed. It appears that lymph nodes and pulmonary metastases responded favorably to IL-2 in 25% and 18%, respectively (Table 4).

As for the dose, all the responders received 10^6 units or more per patient for more than 28 days consecutively (Table 5). There were seven responders in the group receiving daily 10^6 units and three in those receiving daily more than 2×10^6 units. No dose dependency was evident.

Table 4. Efficacy of recombinant interleukin-2 on metastatic organs in renal cell carcinoma

Metastasis	CR+PR	MR+SD+PD	Total	Efficacy (%)
Lung	9	41	50	18.0
Bone		11	11	0.0
Primary lesion	1	9	10	10.0
Lymph node	2	6	8	25.0
Liver		5	5	0.0
Brain		4,	4	0.0
Others		4	4	0.0

CR+PR, responders; *MR+SD+PD*, nonresponders

Table 5. Relationship between the dose of recombinant interleukin-2 and response

Maximum daily dose (U)	CR+PR	MR+SD+PD	Total	Efficacy (%)
0.5×10^6		4	4	0.0
1.0×10^6	7	37	44	15.9
$\geq 2.0 \times 10^6$	3	14	17	17.6

CR+PR, responders; *MR+SD+PD*, nonresponders

Table 6. Effect of previous treatments on response to recombinant interleukin-2

Prior therapy	CR+PR	MR+SD+PD	Total	Efficacy (%)
Nephrectomy	9	46	55	16.4
Chemotherapy	4	17	21	19.0
Immunotherapy	3	24	27	11.1
Radiation		4	4	0.0

CR+PR, responders; *MR+SD+PD*, nonresponders

Relating to prior therapy, there were nine responders among the 55 nephrectomized patients. However, almost the same response rate was observed in patients receiving chemotherapy or immunotherapy prior to IL-2 administration (Table 6).

Table 7 is the summary of the 10 responders. Time requirements for initial response ranged from 2 to 7 weeks. More precisely, the median number of days required for the appearance of effect, 50% shrinkage, and disappearance of lesions was 25.5 (14–47), 47 (28–86), and 114 (88–287), respectively. That of efficacy duration was 244.5 (38–892) in PR and 670 (223–853) in CR. All the responders

Table 7. Summary of the responders

n	Sex and Age	Prior therapy	Sites of responding tumor	Dose (U/day)	Treatment duration (weeks)	Response	Time to response (weeks)	Response duration (months)
1	M 78	Nephrectomy Lumph node (mediastinal)	Lung	1×10^6	32	CR	7	16+
2	M 55	Nephrectomy Interferon	Lung	1×10^6	24	CR	4	25+
3	M 55	Nephrectomy	Lung	1×10^6	8	CR	2	30+
4	M 74	Nephrectomy	Lung	$1 \sim 3 \times 10^6$	23	PR	2	10
5	F 61	Nephrectomy	Lung	$1 \sim 3 \times 10^6$	51	PR	4	11+
6	F 56	Chemotherapy	Kidney Lung	1×10^6	17	PR	4	4
7	M 51	Nephrectomy Chemotherapy	Lung	$1 \sim 3 \times 10^6$	24	PR	6	4+
8	M 58	Nephrectomy Chemotherapy	Lumph node (mediastinal)	1×10^6	8	PR	3	5+
9	M 67	Nephrectomy Chemotherapy	Lung	1×10^6	9	PR	3	1+
10	M 68	Nephrectomy Interferon	Lung	1×10^6	14	PR	4	6+

CR, complete remission; *PR*, partial remission

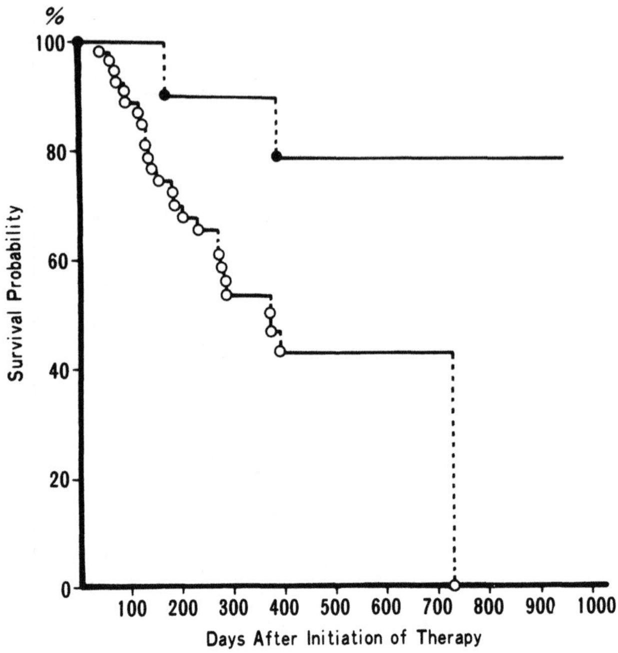

Fig. 1. Comparison of survival rates by Kaplan-Meier's method between the responders and nonresponders. • responders (n = 10); o nonresponders (n = 55)

received prior therapy. Six of them were resistant to interferon or chemotherapeutic agents.

Figure 1 shows the estimated survival probability by Kaplan-Meier's method. It is the most important index in the evaluation of cancer treatment. One and 2 years' survival rates are significantly higher in responders than in nonresponders.

Regarding the change of immunological parameters by IL-2, peripheral white blood cell (WBC) and lymphocytes increased 2 weeks after treatment (Fig. 2).

Both NK and LAK activities were elevated 2 weeks after the consecutive daily administration of IL-2 (Fig. 3).

Study of the lymphocyte subsets showed that the ratios of HLA-DR and IL-2 receptor-positive lymphocytes were increased, although other subsets did not show marked alteration.

IL-2-specific antibody levels were elevated in 2 patients. However, neutralizing antibody was not present, and no clinical effect was observed.

Various side effects are shown in Table 8. Fever, fever with chills, fatigue and headache (influenza-like symptoms) were most frequently seen (84%, 63/75). Then came loss of appetite, nausea, and vomiting (gastrointestinal symptoms) in 38.9% (29/75). However, in no case was it necessary to discontinue the medication. As a serious complication, vascular leak syndrome manifested by water accumulation

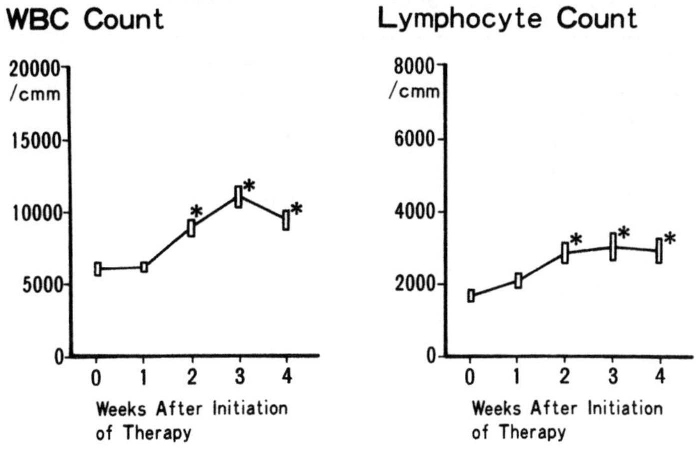

Fig. 2. Effect of recombinant interleukin-2 on white blood cell (*WBC*) and lymphocyte count (mean ± SE). *, $p < 0.05$ (Dunnett's method)

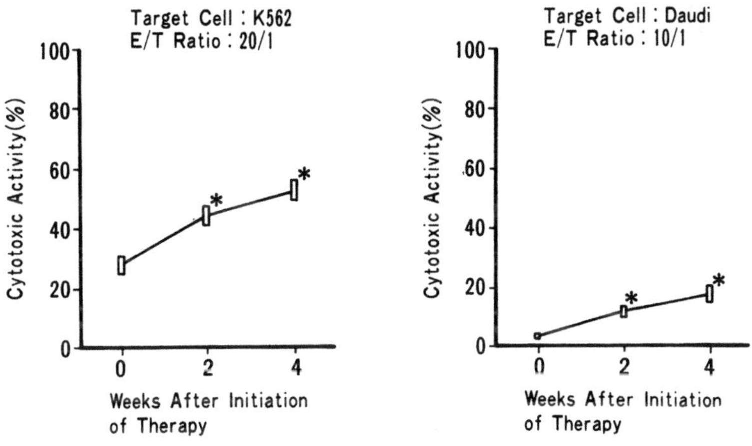

Fig. 3. Effect of recombinant interleukin-2 on lymphocyte activities (mean ± SE). *, $p < 0.05$ (Dunnett's method)

and edema was noted in 5.3% (4/75), and depression and disorientation were seen in 4.0% (3/75). They were all reversible and appeared to be dose-dependent.

Laboratory examination revealed eosinophilia in 57.1% (44/77). No marked bone marrow suppression was present. There was only one patient each with anemia, thrombocytopenia, and hypofibrinogenemia. Two patients with neutropenia were noted. Hepatic and renal dysfunctions were observed in 14.7% (11/75) and 8.0% (6/75), respectively, and were lower than grade 2 according to the WHO grading and occurred mostly in patients receiving more than 2.0×10^6 units per body daily (Table 9).

Table 8. Adverse effects of recombinant interleukin-2

Toxicities	*n*	Percentage
Constitutional		
Fever > 100° F	24	32.0
> 102° F	11	14.6
Chills	15	20.0
Fatigue	13	17.3
Edema	2	2.7
Gastrointestinal		
Anorexia	16	21.3
Nausea and vomiting	8	10.7
Abdominal pain	1	1.3
Abdominal distension	1	1.3
Neurological		
Headache	5	6.7
Depression	2	2.7
Disorientation	1	1.3
Muscles and joints		
Myalgia	3	4.0
Arthralgia	2	2.7
Local irritation	1	1.3

Table 9. Abnormal laboratory data obtained by recombinant interleukin-2 treatment

Toxicities		*n*	Percentage
Hematological:			
Eosinophilia:	> 10%	22	33.8
	> 30%	13	20.0
	> 50%	9	13.8
Leukocytosis:	> 10 000	26	40.0
	> 20 000	3	4.6
Thrombocytopenia:	< 100 000	1	1.5
	< 75 000	1	1.5
Anemia (Hb < 9.5)		6	9.2
Hepatocellular enzyme elevation:			
SGOT > 2.5×N		3	4.6
SGPT > 2.5×N		4	6.2
Alkali phosphatase	> 2.5×N	2	3.1

N, normal value; *SGOT*, serum glutamic-oxaloacetic transaminase; *SGPT*, serum glutamate pyruvate transaminase

In six patients the therapy was discontinued due to side effects including two with hepatic dysfunction, one with renal dysfunction, two with vascular leak syndrome, and one with eosinophilia. They all recovered after discontinuation of the medication.

Figure 4 shows the clinical course of one CR patient. A 55-year-old male underwent right nephrectomy on April 16, 1986 (pT2N0M1V2). Multiple pulmonary metastases ranging from 27 × 20 to 11 × 60 mm were found at the time of initial diagnosis, which were confirmed by fine needle biopsy. On May 6, 1986, IL-2 therapy was initiated. Seven weeks after the therapy, a partial response with 58% shrinkage of metastases was observed. The treatment was discontinued, and the patient was discharged with 8 weeks' administration of daily 10^6 units IL-2. After the discontinuation of the therapy, the remaining lesions continued to shrink. All the metastases disappeared 13 weeks after the initiation. No marked adverse effect was observed.

In Fig. 5A–C, chest X-ray films are compared before, during, and after treatment. They were taken before, 8 weeks, and 13 weeks after the initiation of treatment, respectively.

Discussion

Since the combination of adoptive immunotherapy with IL-2 needs not only a great expense for lymphocyte culture and sophisticated procedures but also intensive care unit monitoring because of severe toxicity with life-threatening impairment of renal, hematologic, pulmonary, and cardiac functions [6–8], IL-2 alone has been used for the treatment of malignancy [4, 5]. Although Rosenberg and his associates [6] reported that an antitumor effect was observed by a large dose (100×10^3/kg, thrice daily) of IL-2, we have seen responders to a small dose treatment (10^6 per body per day) and noted no dose-dependent response. A median of 25.5 days was required before clinical effect was observed. Therefore, at least 4 weeks' administration is necessary to see the effect of IL-2, and it might be desirable to keep patients on it continuously once it proves effective.

A part of the results from trials conducted at the National Cancer Institute [9] is shown in Table 10. Both nonrandomized and randomized trials showed the same response rates with just high-dose IL-2 therapy for renal cell carcinoma (18% and 16%, respectively). However, high-dose IL-2 therapy is always associated with severe toxicity, necessitating intensive monitoring. Various safer methods to give an intermediate dose of IL-2 3×10^6 units/m^2 per day have been investigated with success to a certain degree [10–12]. On the other hand, it should be noted that our trial using low-dose IL-2 revealed similar results without any severe toxicity as reported here.

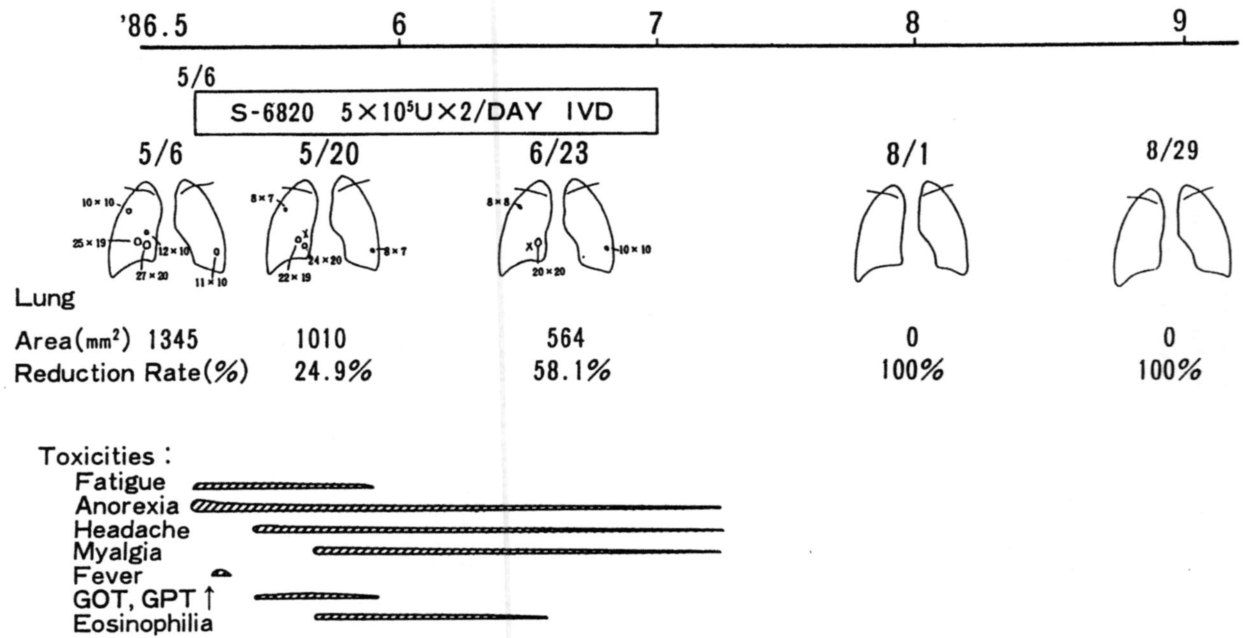

Fig. 4. Prior therapy: nephrectomy (pT2N0M1V2). Clinical course of a 55-year-old male of renal cell carcinoma with pulmonary metastases

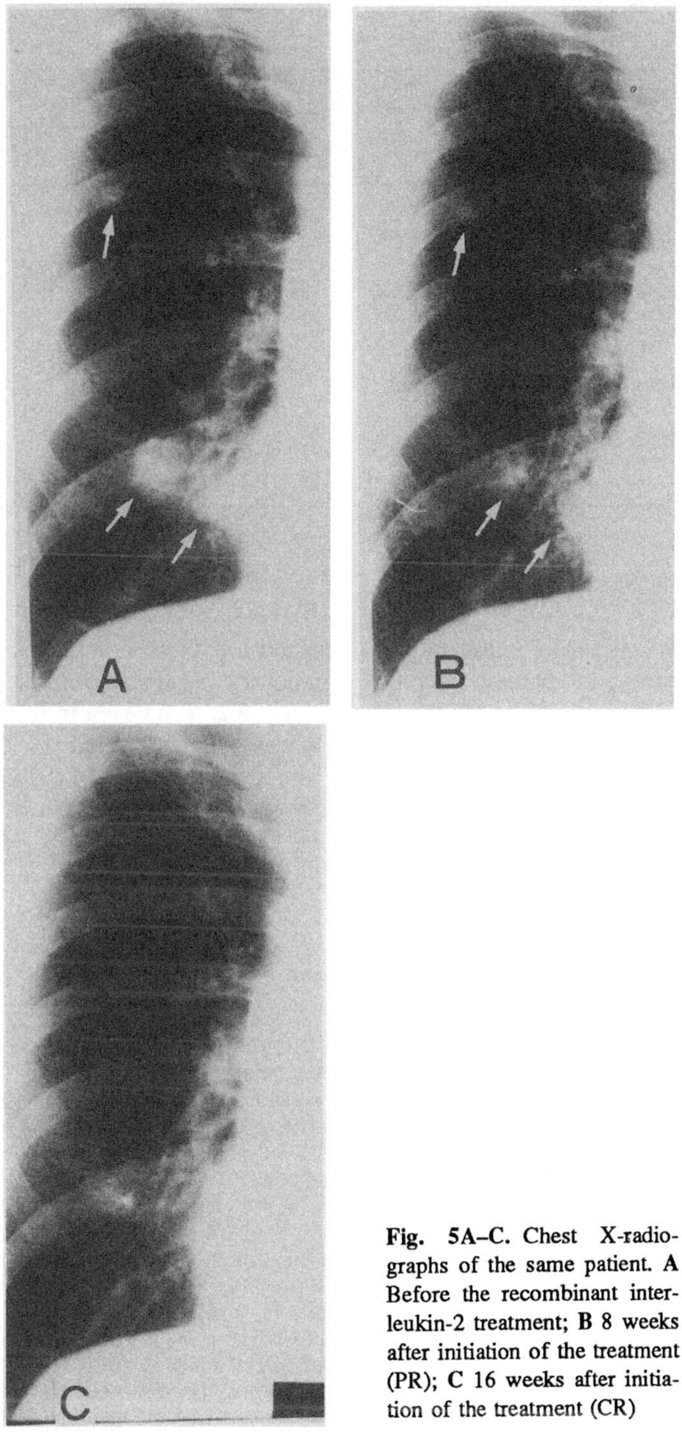

Fig. 5A–C. Chest X-radiographs of the same patient. **A** Before the recombinant interleukin-2 treatment; **B** 8 weeks after initiation of the treatment (PR); **C** 16 weeks after initiation of the treatment (CR)

Table 10. Efficacy of interleukin (IL)-2 with lymphokine-activated killer (LAK) cells and IL-2 alone on advanced cancer [9]

Type of cancer	Type of therapy	*n*	Overall response		Response	
			No.	Percentage	Complete	Partial
			Nonrandomized trial			
Renal carcinoma	IL-2/LAK	54	17	31	7	10
	IL-2	38	7	18	4	3
Melanoma	IL-2/LAK	34	6	18	3	3
	IL-2	23	6	26	0	6
			Randomized trial			
Renal carcinoma	IL-2/Lak	34	10	29	6	4
	IL-2	31	5	16	3	2
Melanoma	IL-2/LAK	16	2	12	2	0
	IL-2	12	4	33	0	4

Conclusions

In conclusion, a low-dose IL-2 treatment is effective for advanced renal cell carcinoma in approximately 15%. Pulmonary and lymph node metastases responded most favorably to the therapy. Efficacy was noted even in patients previously receiving chemotherapy or immunotherapy without marked side effects. We believe that a low-dose IL-2 treatment deserves further trial, and in the future the combination of other biological response modifiers, chemotherapeutic agents, or receptor blockers with low-dose IL-2 should be encouraged to improve further treatment efficacy for advanced renal cell cancer.

References

1. Morgan PA, Ruscetti FW, Gallo R (1976) Selective in vitro growth of T lymphocytes from normal human bone marrows. Science 193:1007–1008
2. Oliver RTD (1988) The clinical potential of interleukin-2. Br J Cancer 58:405–409
3. Rosenberg SA, Lotze MT, Muul LM et al. (1985) Observation on the systemic administration of autologous lymphokine-activated killer cells and recombinant interleukin-2 to patients with metastatic cancer. N Engl J Med 313:1485–1492
4. Rosenberg SA, Lotze T, Mule JJ (1988) New approaches to the immunotherapy of cancer using interleukin-2. Ann Int Med 108:853–864
5. Parkinson DR (1988) Interleukin-2 in cancer therapy. Seminars in Oncology 15 (Suppl 6):10–26
6. Rosenberg SA, Lotze MT, Muul LM et al. (1987) A progress report on the treatment of 157 patients with advanced cancer using lymphokine-activated killer cells and interleukin-2 or high dose interleukin-2 alone. N Eng J Med 316:889–897
7. Fisher RI, Coltman CA, Doroshow JH et al. (1988) Metastatic renal cell cancer treated with interleukin-2 and lymphokine-activated killer cells. Ann Int Med 108:518–523

8. Lotze MT, Chang AE, Seipp CA et al. (1986) High dose recombinant interleukin-2 in the treatment of patients with disseminated cancer: Responses, treatment-related morbidity, and histologic findings. JAMA 256:3117–3124
9. Van Haelst-Pisani CM, Pisani R, Kovach JS (1989) Cancer immunotherapy: Current status of treatment with interleukin-2 and lymphokine-activated killer cells. Mayo Clin Proc 64:451–465
10. Sosman JA, Kohler PC, Hank J et al. (1988) Repetitive weekly cycles of recombinant human interleukin-2: Responses of renal carcinoma with acceptable toxicity. J Natl Cancer Inst 80:60–64
11. Sondel PM, Kohler PC, Hank JA et al. (1988) Recombinant interleukin-2 given by repetitive weekly cycles in patients with cancer: Clinical and immunologic effects. Cancer Res 48:2561–2567
12. Sosman JA, Kohler PC, Hank JA et al. (1988) Repetitive weekly cycles of interleukin-2. II. Clinical and immunologic effects of dose, schedule, and addition of indomethacin. J Natl Cancer Inst 80:1451–1461

Direct Lymphatic Immunotherapy for Metastatic Renal Cell Carcinoma

F. Corrado, C. De Vinci, G. Corrado, and G. Pizza[1]

Rationale of Endolymphatic Immunotherapy

Our first published data in the immunotherapy of urological cancer with Interleukin-2 (IL-2) date from 1984 when we observed for the first time tumor regression of infiltrating bladder cancer caused only by the intralesional injection of IL-2 [1].

The tumor biopsies performed during and at various intervals of time after treatment appeared clearly related both to the intralesional injection of IL-2 and the clinical course of the disease [2]. No adverse clinical side effects or significant general immunological phenomena were observed during the intralesional injection [1, 2].

Continuing our local immunotherapeutic approach we injected some inguinal and supraclavicular metastatic lymph nodes of the patients who had previously undergone nephrectomy for adenocarcinoma of the kidney with low doses of IL-2 (2400 units 3 times in 10 days) and lymphokine-activated killer (LAK) cells (20×10^6 2 times in 3–7 days). We were also surprised to observe the disappearance not only of the injected metastatic lymph nodes but also of the untreated distant ones. We also noted, in some cases, transient splenomegaly.

The histological studies performed on uninjected lymph nodes confirmed the presence of strong inflammatory phenomena and wide necrosis in the metastatic tumor. We also observed in these lymph nodes the presence of helper, cytotoxic-suppressor T lymphocytes and activated T lymphocytes expressing the receptor for IL-2 (alpha-Tac positive cells) with similar percentages. We were also surprised to find about 10% of lymphoid cells expressing the surface marker of thymocytes (CD1+ cells).

What we learned by this experience was the possibility of activating most of the immune competent system simply by injecting lymph nodes with a very small amount of IL-2, 2000–5000 U, and a few million LAK cells.

The following step was relatively simple. We decided to evaluate whether or not the direct injection of IL-2 and LAK cells into the main external lymphatics of the feet could be of help in "activating" the immune system and controlling neoplastic growth.

[1] 1st Division of Urology and Experimental Service of Urology, M. Malpighi Hospital, Via P. Palagi, 9, 40138 Bologna, Italy

F.M.J. Debruyne et al. (Eds.)
Immunotherapy of Renal Cell Carcinoma

Table 1. Endolymphatic protocol treatment with interleukin-2 in metatatic renal cancer

Timing	Monthly injection
Route	Lymphatics of the feet
IL-2 dose	10 000 U in 10 ml saline
LAK cells	16+/–7 $\times 10^6$ autologous
Duration of injection	30–45 min
Duration of treatment	6 months after complete remission or persistence of disease
Premedication	10 mg chlorpheniramine maleate 30 min before injection

Table 2. Immunological effects in vitro: percentage variation of peripheral blood lymphocyte subsets from renal cancer patients ($n = 8$) after 72 h incubation with 20 U interleukin (IL)-2

	Monocytes	HLA-DR	CD4	CD8	CD16	CD4/CD8
Control	17	21	21	23	19	1.31
SD	10	10	7	14	7	1.49
20 U IL-2	31	29	33	28	32	1.36
SD	15	10	10	11	9	0.74
Student's t	0.016	0.006	0.001	NS	0.003	NS
Wilcoxon	0.05	0.01	0.01	NS	0.01	NS

NS, not significant; *HLA-DR*, D related histocompatibility antigens; *CD*, cluster designation antigen; *SD*, standard deviation

Treatment Protocol

Table 1 shows the protocol we decided on in our pretrial study, having previously assessed that injections via the lymphatics of 30 000 units of our IL-2 was accompanied in most cases by undesired clinical side effects (Table 1).

We also observed that 20 units represented the lowest dose necessary for obtaining significant modification of surface lymphoid markers in vitro, so we chose this concentration for therapeutic purposes.

In Vitro Results

Table 2 shows the mean percentage variation observed in eight patients with renal cancer before the cells and IL-2 were injected into the lymphatics. We observed a statistically significant increase in the percentage of monocytes and lymphocytes expressing HLA-DR antigens and CD4+ and CD16+. No significant changes were observed for CD8+.

Table 3. Immunological effects in vivo: percentage variations of peripheral blood lymphocyte membrane surface markers in 13 patients with metastatic renal cell cancer treated with IL-2 and LAK cells. Values were obtained immediately before injection and 24 h after IL-2 administration

μl	Leucocytes	Lymphocytes	CD3	CD4	CD8	Alpha-Tac
Before	7161	1734	953	774	855	631
SD	3796	664	616	467	425	493
After IL-2 and LAK	8380	2311	1478	1191	1308	979
SD	4016	737	728	726	688	520
Student's *t*	NS	0.001	0.003	0.001	0.01	0.04
Wilcoxon	NS	0.01	0.01	0.05	0.02	NS
N° >/N° <	6/6	7/5	10/2	9/4	10/3	9/3
N° </N° >	0/12	0/12	0/12	1/12	1/12	1/11
Chi square	NS	0.03	0.001	0.001	0.0004	0.001

> = 1 *SD* increase; < = 1 *SD* diminuition; *IL-2*, interleukin-2;
LAK, lymphokine-activated killer. *N°*, number of patients with 1 SD variation

Table 4. Immunological effects in vivo: peripheral blood lymphocyte mitogen reactivity of 9 patients with metastatic renal cell cancer treated with IL-2 and LAK cells. Values were obtained immediately before and 24 h after the second administration

	Control	PHA 0.1 μl	PHA 1 μl	PHA 3 μl	ConA 30 μl
Before	3796	38958	102425	101061	40233
SD	1924	26345	71235	72384	41182
After IL-2 and LAK	3817	58165	127790	107164	52476
SD	1564	53747	73383	68791	42315
Student's *t*	NS	NS	NS	NS	NS
Wilcoxon	NS	NS (0.1)	NS	NS	NS (0.1)
N° >/N° <	3/6	5/4	6/3	6/3	6/3
N° </N° >	4/5	1/8	1/8	2/7	1/8
Chi square	NS	NS	0.02	NS	0.02

> = 1 *SD* increase; < = 1 *SD* diminuition; *IL-2*, interleukin-2;
LAK, lymphokine-activated killer; *PHA*, phytohemagglutinin; *ConA*, concanavalin A

Table 3 depicts the immunological effects observed in vivo on peripheral blood lymphocyte (PBL) subsets of the 13 patients with metastatic renal cancer studied. 24 h after IL-2 and LAK cells administration we noticed in 6 patients that the neutrophils had increased, but only in a few of them was this significant. In contrast, in most patients we found a significant increase of total PBL, CD3+, CD4+, CD8+, and alpha-Tac expressing cell surface antigens.

Table 5. Endolymphatic administration of interleukin (IL)-2 (10 ml) and lymphokine-activated killer (LAK) cells (53×10^6) in patients with metastatic renal cancer: peripheral blood cellular kinetics. Before, during and at intervol time after injection

	Red blood cells ($\times 10^6$)	Leucocytes	Neutrophiles	Lymphocytes	Monocytes	Eosinophils	Basophils	Platelets ($\times 10^3$)
Before	3.62	3380	1590	640	260	810	80	139
During	3.53	3370	1520	690	270	800	60	146
After: 30 min	3.41	3260	1590	590	290	680	70	149
60 min	3.68	890[b]	650[b]	650	100[b]	390[b]	30[b]	11[b, c]
90 min	3.36	3790	2230[a]	430[b]	240	740	70	142
2 h	3.78	5780[a]	4120[a]	530	330	670	90	77[b, d]
3 h	3.71	6410[a]	4610[a]	520	500[a]	650	90	154
4 h	3.32	5830[a]	4160[a]	560	420[a]	560[b]	70	137
5 h	3.45	6580[a]	5000[a]	500	460[a]	480[b]	50[b]	145
6 h	3.47	6450[a]	4970[a]	490	410[a]	440[b]	60	149
10 h	3.33	5550[a]	3930[a]	560	410[a]	540[b]	70	139
24 h	3.72	7160[a]	5650[a]	690	520[a]	180[b]	80	181[a]
48 h	nt	nt	nt	nt	nt	nt	nt	nt

[a] > 30%
[b] < 30%
[c] platelet clumps
[d] clots

The effects on mitogen triggering are depicted in Table 4. In 6 out of 9 patients we noticed a significant increase of both phytohemagglutinin (PHA) and concanavalin A (ConA) lymphocyte stimulation. When the data of all patients were pooled no statistically significant difference could be found because of the high variability of the individual responses.

Regarding the timing of appearance in the blood of the cellular kinetic variations, Table 5 depicts the typical pattern. A rapid increase of neutrophils, lymphocytes, monocytes, and eosinophils, sometimes followed immediately by a slight or dramatic decrease of these values, can be observed in the first few hours after IL-2 and LAK cell administration. The increased values remained generally stable for 2–4 days and progressively returned to the previous values in 5–6 days.

Patient Population and Follow-up

We treated 17 patients (aged 18–79 years) with renal cell carcinoma suffering from 2–12 multiple metastases. They had already undergone surgical removal of the primary tumor 6–30 months before treatment, and all were suffering from progressive disease at the start of immunotherapy. The histological grade of the primary tumors were 7 G2 and 10 G3. Ten patients also had multiorgan involvement. Seven patients underwent adjuvant complementary telecobalt radiation treatment.

Clinical side effects (type and percentage are depicted in Table 6) were minimal and did not require hospitalization in the intensive care unit in any of the patients treated. Most of our patients were treated as outpatients.

Table 7 shows the tumor indicator site chosen according to the possibility of measuring the pertinent diameters of the lesions. Clinical objective response, its duration, the number of treatments, the follow-up, and the status of the individual patients are also reported. The evaluation of the response was performed in accordance with standard criteria.

The mean duration of the follow-up was 12+/–9 months (ranging from 2 to 30) with 4.5+/–2.4 treatment cycles (ranging from 2 to 10).

Table 6. Clinical side effects in 17 patients with metastatic renal cancer treated by the endolymphatic route

Chills	26%
Fever (less than 38°C)	42%
Nausea and vomiting	26%
Cutaneous rash	10%
Hypotension (> 20 mmHg)	7%
Pain (inguinal lymph nodes)	10%

Table 7. Individual results of treatment of renal metastatic cancer with interleukin (IL)-2 and lymphokine-activated killer (LAK) cells endolymphatically administered in 17 patients

Patients	Indicator site	Treatment cycles	Clinical response	Other site	Follow-up (months)	Status
SI[a]	Kidney	6	SD (12)	–	15	Alive
CA	LFN	6	CR (6)/PROG	PR (bone)	18	Alive
MA	Lung	8	SD (6)/PROG	–	18	Alive
CI 1st	Med lung	6	MR (6)/PROG	CR (ing.lfn)[c]	16	Alive
CI 2nd	Med lung	2	PR (2)	–	2	Alive
FA	LFN[b]	6	CR (6)	PROG	9	Dead
RA	Lung	6	PR (12)	PROG (bone)	26	Dead
ZU	Lung	3	PROG	–	3	Dead
BO	Lung	7	CR (26)	–	30	Alive
LA	Mediastinum	2	PR (6)/PROG	PROG (liver, brain)	15	Dead
CH	Lung	8	PROG	–	8	Alive
FE	Pleura	2	SD (2)	–	2	Alive
RI	Lung	2	PROG	–	2	Dead
CO	Lung	2	PROG	–	2	Dead
BE	Lung	4	PROG	–	4	Dead
GO	Lung	3	PROG	PROG (bone)	3	Alive
SA	Mediastinum	2	SD (4)	SD	4	Alive
FA[a]	Kidney	2	SD (2)	–	2	Alive

LFN, lymphnodes; *Med lung*, mediastinum and lung; *ing. lfn*, inguinal lymphnodes; *CR*, complete response (100%); *PR*, partial response (> 50%); *MR*, minor response (> 25% and < 50%); *SD*, stable disease; *PROG*, progression (> 25%).

[a] primary tumor

[b] also intralesional injection

[c] *TCT* also

Clinical Results

Table 8 depicts the percentages and duration of the different clinical responses in both the indicator and other sites. In three patients we noticed both complete response (duration 6, 6, and 26 months); in three partial response (duration 2, 12, and 6 months); in one, minor response (duration 6 months); in five stable disease (duration, 2, 2, 4, 8, 12 months); and in six, progression. Positive clinical responses were observed in 7 out of 17 patients (41%), stabilization of the disease in 5 (29%), and progression in 6 (35%) (Table 9).

Five out of seven (71%) patients who experienced a positive clinical response afterwards had progression of the disease, and three of them (60%) died 6, 15, and 26 months after the beginning of immunotherapy (Table 9). It is worth noting here that the mean survival, 15 months, is higher than that seen in patients treated

Table 8. Clinical results for patients with renal metastatic cancer treated with interleukin (IL)-2 and lymphokine-activted killer (LAK) cells endolymphatically administered

	Clinical response						Alive/ dead
	Complete	Partial	Minor disease	Stable	Mixed[a]	Pro- gression	
Indicator site ($n = 17$)	3	3	1	5	0	6	
Duration (months)	6,6,26	2,12,6	6	8,12,1,4,2			10/7
Other site ($n = 6$)	1	1	0	0	1	4	
Duration (months)	12						

[a] Mixed regression and progression at the same time at different sites

Table 9. Clinical results at the indicator sites in treatment with interleukin (IL)-2 and lymphokine-activated killer (LAK) cells endolymphatically administered in patients with metastatic renal cancer

	CR+PR+MR	Stable	Progression	Dead
Patients ($n = 17$)	7 (41%)	5 (29%)	6 (35%)	
CR+PR+MR ($n = 7$)			5 (71%) →	3/5 (60%)
Months from the beginning of immunotherapy to death				6,26,15 ($\bar{x} = 15$)

C, complete; *P*, partial; *M*, minor; *R*, regression

conventionally or not treated at all. In fact, the mean survival for untreated patients is 9 months from the diagnosis of metastasis. In addition, the mean survival of patients treated with immunotherapy is calculated from the beginning of treatment and not from the time of appearance of metastasis.

While searching for the possible existence of markers able to predict the response to IL-2 immunotherapy we wanted to see whether tumor necrosis factor (TNF) could be considered to be involved (8–9). Serum samples were drawn from seven patients both during and immediately after IL-2 and LAK administration as shown in Table 10 where data obtained in the first four patients are reported.

When TNF activity is induced, its appearance or increase in serum is immediate, starting even during IL-2 injection or after 15–30 min and lasting for 24–48 h with some variations.

The preliminary data show mild increase or appearance of TNF in four patients who experienced complete tumor regression (2), stable disease (1), or progression (1). In contrast, in the remaining three in whom no TNF activity was induced in the serum, we observed rapid progressive disease (Table 10).

Table 10. Correlations between tumor necrosis factor (TNF) appearance or increase (> 10 pg/ml) in sera of patients with metastatic renal cancer treated by endolymphatic administration of interleukin-2 and lymphokine-activated killer cells

Patients	TNF increase	Clinical response
ZUL	No	Progression
FAC	Yes	Complete regression
BEN	No	Progression
MAS	No	Progression
CAL	Yes	Complete regression
CHI	Yes	Progression
FER	Yes	Stable disease

Conclusions

From the data presented we can draw the following conclusions:

1. The use of IL-2 significantly increases the lymphoid markers when incubated in vitro even at low concentration (20 U) with PBL both of normal and metastatic RCC patients, overall monocytes, HLA-DR, CD4+, CD16+ cells.
2. The endolymphatic administration of IL-2 significantly increases the peripheral blood lymphoid marker subsets in metastatic RCC patients: overall total lymphocytes, CD3+, CD4+, CD8+, and alpha-Tac antigen positive cells; in addition, in half of the patients, lymphoid mitogen triggering (PHA-P and ConA) also appears to be significantly increased.
3. Confirming observations of other workers using different administration routes (3, 4), no correlations can be established between in vitro and in vivo immunological modifications of the parameters studied and the clinical response in RCC patients (5); in addition, despite our preliminary observations, no clear correlations were established between variations of TNF levels of sera and clinical course.
4. We confirm the observations of other workers who used the PB administration route; in fact 41% (7 out of 17) of our metastatic RCC patients, treated endolymphatically, experienced a positive clinical response (3, 4). Considering the scarce clinical adverse side effects the results of our pretrial study appear, in our opinion, encouraging.

Of course, our results, although encouraging, must be considered preliminary. Regarding the similar results obtained by other workers using recombinant IL-2 with a larger number of patients treated with much higher doses injected into the bloodstream, no comparison is possible (3–7). In fact, the IL-2 that we produce ourselves from a gibbon lymphoblastoid cell line is a native one, and its gene DNA coding sequence presents 99% homology with the human gene. In contrast, recombinant

IL-2 is not glycosylated. In addition, the methods for evaluating the biological activity are different: we use PHA-activated human lymphoblast growth in IL-2 conditioned medium, others use murine T cell line [1].

Only common treatment protocols using both interleukins and the same administration route can give some indication of any analogy in the results.

References

1. Pizza G, Severini G, Menniti D, De Vinci C, Corrado F (1984) Tumour regression after intralesional injection of interleukin-2 (IL-2) in bladder cancer: preliminary report. Int J Cancer 34:359–367
2. Pizza G, Bertoni F, Casanova S, De Vinci C, Corrado F (1987) Interleukin-2 in the treatment of infiltrating bladder cancer. J Exp Pathol 3:525–531
3. Rosenberg SA, Lotze MT, Muul LM et al. (1985) Observations on the systemic administration of autologous lymphokine-activated killer cells and recombinant interleukin-2 to patients with metastatic cancer. N Engl J Med 313:1485–1492
4. Rosenberg AS, Lotze M, Muul L et al. (1987) A progress report on the treatment of 157 patients with advanced cancer using lymphokine-activated killer cells and interleukin-2 or high-dose interleukin-2 alone. N Engl J Med 316:889–897
5. Belldegrun A, Uppenkamp I, Rosenberg S (1988) Anti tumour reactivity of human lymphokine activated killer (LAK) cells against fresh and cultured preparations of renal cell cancer. J Urol 139:150–155
6. Fisher RI, Coltman CA, Doroshow JH et al. (1988) Metastatic renal cancer treated with interleukin-2 and lymphokine activated killer cells. Ann Int Med 108:518–552
7. Sosman JA, Kohller PC, Hank J et al. (1988) Repetitive weekly cycles of recombinant human interleukin-2: responses of renal carcinoma with acceptable toxicity. J Natl Cancer Inst 80:60–63
8. Ruggiero V, Latham K, Baglioni C (1987) Cytostatic and cytotoxic activity of tumour necrosis factor on human cancer cells. J Immunol 138:2711–2717
9. Heicappel R, Naito S, Ichinose Y et al. (1987) Cytostatic and cytolytic effects of human recombinant tumour necrosis factor on human renal cell carcinoma cell lines derived from a single surgical specimen. J Immunol 138:1634–1640

Combination Therapy of Renal Cell Carcinoma with Interleukin-2 and Interferon Alpha: The Cleveland Clinic Experience

G.T. Budd, J. Sergi, J. Finke, B. Barna, J. Boyett, S. Medendorp, S. Murthy, R. Tubbs, V. Gibson, J.E. Pontes, and R.M. Bukowski [1]

Introduction

Interleukin-2 (IL-2) and interferon alpha (IFNα) are immunomodulatory cytokines which can now be produced in bulk using recombinant DNA techniques. The availability of these agents has rejuvenated the field of cancer immunotherapy, and clinical trials utilizing them have been performed with a variety of malignancies. Because renal cell carcinoma (RCC) is resistant to traditional systemic therapies and because earlier immunotherapy trials had suggested that it may be susceptible to immunologic therapy, this tumor system has been among the most intensively studied in trials investigating the therapeutic potential of these new biologic agents.

Interferon Alpha

Recombinant human IFNα (rHuIFNα2a) is a 19 264 dalton MW glycoprotein composed of 165 amino acids. It is produced using recombinant DNA techniques and purified by affinity chromatography. IFNα is directly cytotoxic or cytostatic for some cancer cells and may augment the immunogenicity of malignant cells by enhancing the expression of histocompatibility and tumor-associated antigens [1–5]. Immunologic effects of IFNα include the augmentation of natural killer (NK) and cytolytic T-cell cytotoxicity [6–10].

While IFNα is highly active in the therapy of hairy cell leukemia, its usefulness as a therapeutic agent for solid tumors is modest; in RCC, the response rate is approximately 15% [1].

Interleukin-2

IL-2 is a lymphokine which is secreted by lymphocytes. Recombinant IL-2 (rIL-2) is produced in an *E. coli* expression vector from a gene cloned from a human lymphoblastoid T-cell line (Jurkat lymphoma). The nonglycosylated recombinant

[1] The Cleveland Clinic Foundation, One Clinic Center, 9500 Euclid Avenue, Cleveland, OH 44195, USA

F.M.J. Debruyne et al. (Eds.)
Immunotherapy of Renal Cell Carcinoma

material produced by Hoffman-La Roche is approximately 95% pure, with a specific activity of approximately 1.5×10^7 U/mg protein.

IL-2 exerts profound effects on the immune system, acting to induce and support T-cell growth, induce helper T-cell function, activate antigen-specific cytotoxic T lymphocytes, augment NK activity, and induce lymphokine-activated killer (LAK) cell activity [11–13].

As a single agent or as part of adoptive immunotherapy programs using LAK cells generated from peripheral blood, IL-2 therapy produces objective antitumor effects in 9%–26% of patients with metastatic RCC [14, 15].

Preclinical Studies of Combination Therapy with IL-2 and IFNα

Because lymphokines act in concert in vivo, it might be anticipated that some combinations of cytokines will prove significantly more active than their single agent constituents in terms of specific immune effects, such as the antitumor response. In a murine system, IL-2 and IFNαA/D were synergistic in their effects on NK-cell activity [16]. In vivo studies of these agents have demonstrated that the combination is more active in terms of antitumor effect than are the single component lymphokines [17, 18].

Clinical Trials of rIL-2 and rHuIFNα2a at the Cleveland Clinic Foundation

Based upon the preclinical studies described above, a series of phase I studies were performed at the Cleveland Clinic Foundation. Successive groups of 4–6 patients were treated with sequentially higher doses of the cytokines. All patients suffered from a metastatic malignancy refractory to conventional therapy or malignancy for which no standard therapy exists, had good performance status (0–1 by ECOG or SWOG criteria), and had satisfactory major organ function.

In the first phase I trial, 55 patients received rIL-2 0.1, 0.5, or 2.0×10^6 U/m^2 by i.v. bolus injection on Mondays, Wednesdays, and Fridays for 4 consecutive weeks in conjunction with rHuIFNα2a at doses of 0, 0.1, 1.0, or 10.0×10^6 U/m^2 i.m. on Mondays, Wednesdays, or Fridays. Neutrophil nadirs of < 1000/mm^3 (1.0×10^9/l) were produced in 3/6 patients treated at the highest doses of the two cytokines (rIL-2, 2.0×10^6 U/m^2 and rHuIFNα2a, 10.0×10^6 U/m^2), defining the maximum tolerated dose according to conventional criteria [19].

Because the nonhematologic toxicity was mild and the rapidly reversible neutropenia observed was not associated with any infectious complications, the definitions of unacceptable toxicity were modified, and dose escalation continued. Currently, rIL-2 22.0×10^6 U/m^2 i.v. and rHuIFNα2a 10.0×10^6 U/m^2 i.m. are being given together thrice weekly. At these higher doses, most patients develop symptomatic hypotension requiring support with the vasopressor phenylephrine. Reversible elevations of serum creatinine and transaminases have been produced, and occasional patients suffered confusion, respiratory distress, oliguria, or cardiac arrhythmia. Most patients experienced tolerable skin rash and diarrhea, while all patients developed fever, chills, nausea, and fatigue. These toxicities are formidable but can be managed by knowledgeable medical and nursing staff [20].

Because infusion schedules of IL-2 seem to have more profound effects on some immune parameters and because continuous infusion schedules more closely mimic the pharmacokinetics of the intraperitoneal and subcutaneous administration methods used in preclinical model systems, we conducted a phase I trial of rIL-2 by continuous infusion for 120 h in conjunction with thrice weekly IFNα. Treatment was given for 4 consecutive weeks. IL-2 3.0×10^6 U/m^2 every 24 h was tolerable when combined with doses of rHuIFNα2a of 5.0 and 10.0×10^6 U/m^2, but unacceptable hepatic, pulmonary, and central nervous system toxicities were produced by the combination of rIL-2 4.5×10^6 U/m^2 every 24 h and IFNα 5.0×10^2 U/m^2 i.m. [21].

In addition to these phase I trials, the Cleveland Clinic Foundation participated in a multicenter trial of IL-2 3.0×10^6 U/m^2 per 24 h for 4 consecutive days in conjunction with IFNα 5.0×10^6 U/m^2 i.m. for 4 consecutive days. These treatments were administered weekly for 4 consecutive weeks, followed by a 2-week rest period. This dose schedule was based on a phase I trial reported by Lee and colleagues [22]. At the Cleveland Clinic, we treated a total of 11 patients with metastatic RCC as a part of this multicenter phase II trial; 1 complete and 3 partial responses have been observed. Of 12 patients with RCC treated in the low-dose phase I bolus schedule trial, 1 has responded, while 2/17 treated with high-dose rIL-2 and rHuIFNα2a by a bolus schedule have responded. Some 3/7 patients with RCC treated as a part of the phase I infusion schedule trial have shown objective responses to therapy. Some of these responses have been of particular clinical significance, with one patient remaining free of disease more than 12 months after resection of the material remaining after a nearly complete response of bulky disease to combination cytokine therapy. These results are summarized in Table 1.

Table 1. Response to interleukin-2 plus recombinant human interferon alpha-2a therapy in metastatic renal cell carcinoma

Dose schedule	No. of renal cell cancer patients treated	Complete responses	Partial responses	Response rate
Lowdose bolus	12	0	1	0.08
Highdose bolus	17	0	2	0.12
Infusion, phase I	7	0	3	0.43
Infusion, phase II	11	1	3	0.36
Bolus, overall	29	0	3	0.10
Infusion, overall	18	1	6	0.39

Immunologic Effects of Therapy with rIL-2 plus rHuIFNα2a

As might be expected from their single agent activities, IL-2 and IFNα in combination exert significant effects on the immune system. Most patients treated as a part of the clinical trials described above have undergone serial studies of selected immunologic parameters prior to and during therapy. Therapy with rIL-2 and rHuIFNα2a is associated with a marked increase in NK activity in the peripheral blood; LAK activity is also generated. The magnitude of this augmentation of NK activity seems to be positively related to the dose of IL-2. In the initial bolus trial, in which the widest range of IFNα doses was studied, the greatest degree of augmentation of NK activity seemed to be at a low dose of IFNα, 0.1×10^6 U/m^2 [19]. These dose-effect relationships are similar to those observed with single-agent cytokine therapy [23, 24]. No definite correlations between either NK or LAK activity and antitumor effect have been able to be demonstrated [19, 21].

Studies of the phenotypic distribution of peripheral blood lymphocytes have shown an increase in the number of CD56$^+$ (leu19$^+$) lymphocytes as a consequence of IL-2 and IFNα therapy [21]; this subset has been shown to harbor most of the NK and LAK activity [25].

The total number of T cells (CD3$^+$) in the peripheral blood seems to decrease during the first week of rIL-2 plus rHuIFNα2a therapy, followed by a recovery to baseline levels. After the first week, the number of activated T cells (CD3+HLA-DR+CD25- and CD3+HLA-DR+CD25+) increases in the peripheral blood [21].

Because the lymphocytes infiltrating tumors are most proximate to the tumor cells, these lymphocytes are of major interest. Interestingly, when one semiquantitatively grades the intensity of infiltration from 0-trace to 4+, that with CD56+ lymphocytes is 0, trace, or 1+, both prior to and with rIL-2 plus rHuIFNα2a therapy. This dichotomy of effects on peripheral blood and tumor-infiltrating lymphocytes calls into question the relevance of observations based upon changes in the peripheral blood alone. The majority of tumor-infiltrating lymphocytes are CD3+, and the intensity of infiltration with CD3+ lymphocytes, both prior to and with therapy, is positively correlated with the intensity of human leukocyte antigen (HLA-DR) expression [26]. This relationship has also been described by others for patients treated with IL-2-based regimens [27].

Conclusions

Overall, 10/47 patients with RCC have responded to rIL-2 and rHuIFNα2a therapy, for a major response rate of 21%. These preliminary studies would suggest that the infusion schedule of rIL-2, when given with rHuIFNα2a, is superior to the bolus schedule. The response rate was 7/18 (39%, 95% Confidence Interval (CI) 17%–61%) for patients treated with infusion rIL-2 as compared with 3/29 (10%, 95% CI 0%–22%) for patients treated with bolus schedule rIL-2. It must be remembered, however, that all patients treated with infusion rIL-2 in our studies received a dose of 3.0×10^6 U/m^2 per 24 h, the maximum tolerated dose that can be given by continuous infusion with rHuIFNα2a 5–10 $\times 10^6$ U/m^2. The vast majority of patients treated with bolus schedule rIL-2, on the other hand, were treated with doses that were less than the maximum tolerated dose. Thus, the influences of schedule and dose cannot be distinguished by our studies.

Phase II trials of this combination in this disease are warranted, as are further immunologic studies in treated patients. Only by elucidation of the mechanisms by which antitumor effects are mediated can the rational development of recombination cytokine therapy proceed.

References

1. Goldstein D, Laszlo J (1986) Interferon therapy in cancer: from imaginon to interferon. Cancer Res 46:4315–4329
2. Lindahl P, Leary P, Gresser I (1972) Enhancement by interferon of the specific cytotoxicity of sensitized lymphocytes. Proc Natl Acad Sci USA 69:721–725
3. Murray JL, Rosenblum MG et al. (1986) Differential in vitro effects of alpha recombinant interferon and gamma recombinant interferon on the expression of melanoma-eassociated antigens (MAA) P97 and 240 Kd on melanoma cell line Ts294. Proc Natl Acad Sci USA 27:313
4. Giacomini P, Aguzzi A, Pestka S et al. (1984) Modulation by recombinant DNA leukocyte (alpha) and fibroblast (beta) interferons of the expression and shedding of HLA and tumor-associated antigens by human melanoma cells. J Immunol 133:1649–1655
5. Rosenblum MG, Lamki LM, Murray JL et al. (1988) Interferon-induced changes in pharmacokinetics and tumor uptake of ^{111}In-labelled antimelanoma antibody 96.5 in melanoma patients. J Natl Cancer Inst 80:160–165
6. Herberman RB, Ortaldo JR, Mantovani A et al. (1982) Effect of human recombinant interferon on cytotoxic activity of natural killer (NK) cells and monocytes. Cell Immunol 67:160–167
7. Brunda RB, Rosenbaum D (1934) Modulation of murine natural killer cell activity in vitro and in vivo by recombinant human interferons. Cancer Res 44:597–601
8. Brunda MJ, Rosenbaum D, Stern L (1984) Inhibition of experimentally-induced metastases by recombinant alpha interferon: correlation between the modulatory effect of interferon treatment on natural killer cell activity and inhibition of metastses. Int J Cancer 24:421–426
9. Suzuki R, Suzuki S, Ebina N, Kumagai K (1985) Suppression of alloimmune cytotoxic T lymphocyte (CTL) generation by depletion of NK cells and restoration by interferon and/or interleukin 2. J Immunol 134:2139–2148
10. Herberman RB (1980) Natural cell mediated immunity against tumors. Academic Press, New York
11. Henney CS, Huribayashi K, Kern DE, Gillis S (1981) Interleukin-2 augments natural keller cell activity. Nature 291:335–338
12. Stotter H, Rude E, Wagner H (1980) T cell factor (interleukin 2) allows in vivo induction of T helper cells against heterologous erythrocytes in athymic (nu/nu) mice. Eur J Immunol 10:719–722
13. Errard F, Corthesy P, Nabhol M et al. (1985) Interleukin-2 is both necessary and sufficient for the growth and differentiation of lectin-stimulated cytolytic T lymphocyte precursors. J Immunol 134:1644–1651

14. Fisher RI, Coltman CA, Doroshow JH et al. (1988) Metastatic renal cancer treated with interleukin-2 and lymphokine-activated killer cells. A phase II clinical trial. Ann Intern Med 108:518–523
15. Bukowski RM, Goodman P, Crawford ED et al. (1989) Phase II evaluation of recombinant interleukin-2 (rIL-2) in metastatic renal cell carcinoma (RCC): SWOG 8617. Proc ASCO 8:143
16. Brunda MJ, Tarnowski D, Davatelis V (1986) Interaction of recombinant interferons with recombinant interleukin-2: differential effects on natural killer cell activity and interleukin-2 activated killer cells. Int J Cancer 37:797–793
17. Chikkala NF, Lewis I, Ulchaker, Finke JH et al. (1990) Interactive effects of α-interferon A/D and interleukin 2 on murine lymphokine-activated killer activity: analysis at the effector and precursor level. Cancer Res 50:1176–1182
18. Iigo M, Sakurai M, Tamura T et al. (1988) In vivo antitumor activity of multiple injections of recombinant interleukin 2, alone and in combination with three different types of recombinant interferon, on various syngeneic murine tumors. Cancer Res 48:260–264
19. Budd GT, Osgood B, Barna B et al. (1989) Phase I clinical trial of interleukin 2 and α-interferon: toxicity and immunologic effects. Cancer Res 49:6432–6436
20. Budd GT, Sergi J, Barna B et al. (1989) Phase I trial of interleukin-2 (rIL-2) and INFα (rHuIFNα2a) in human malignancy. Proc Natl Acad Sci USA 30:362
21. McKeever S, Funke J, Murthy S et al. (1989) Phase 1a/1b trial of high dose continuous infusion (CI) interleukin-2 (rIL-2) and interferon (rHuIFNα2a): preliminary clinical and laboratory results. Proc Am Assoc Cancer Res 30:238
22. Lee KH, Talpaz M, Rohberg JM et al. (1989) Concimitant administration of recombinant human interleukin-2 and recombinant interferon alpha-2A in cancer patients: a phase I study. J Clin Oncol 7:1726–1732
23. Edwards BS, Hawkins MJ, Borden EC (1984) Comparative in vivo and in vitro activation of human natural killer cells by recombinant α-interferons differing in antiviral activity. Cancer Res 44:3135–3139
24. Edwards BS, Merritt JA; Fuhlbrigge RC, Borden EC (1985) Low doses of interferon alpha result in more effective clinical natural killer cell activation. J Clin Invest 75:1908–1913
25. Phillips JH, Gemlo BT, Myers WW et al. (1987) In vivo and in vitro activation of natural killer cells in advanced cancer patients undergoing combined recombinant interleukin-2 and LAK cell therapy. J Clin Oncol 5:1933–1941
26. Tubbs R, Budd GT, Finke J et al. (1990) Cellular infiltrates in tumor specimens from patients treated with cytokines and adoptive cellular therapy. Proc Am Assoc Cancer Res 31:175
27. Rubin JT, Elwood LJ, Rosenberg SA, Lotze MT (1989) Immunohistochemical correlates of response to recombinant interleukin-2 based immunotherapy in humans. Cancer Res 49:7086–7092

Tumor Infiltrating Lymphocytes in Human Renal Cell Carcinoma: Adoptive Immunotherapy and Characterization of Interleukin-2 Expanded Tumor-Infiltrating Lymphocytes

J. Finke, S. Murthy, J. Alexander, P. Rayman, R. Tubbs, J.E. Pontes, J. Sergi, and R.M. Bukowski [1]

Introduction

Tumor-infiltrating lymphocytes (TILs) appear to represent part of the host immune response to the tumor and may contain an enriched population of cells with reactivity to the autologous tumor [1–4]. Most of the infiltrating cells are T lymphocytes, with the number of $CD8^+$ cells being greater than $CD4^+$ cells [1–7]. Several human solid tumors have been reported to contain an increased frequency of cytotoxic precursors against autologous tumor when compared with peripheral blood lymphocytes [8]. In addition, recent studies have shown that TILs were therapeutically more potent than interleukin (IL)-2-activated spleen cells in several murine tumor models [9, 10].

Based on the preclinical studies in animal models, phase I/II trials have been conducted with human TILs [11–13]. Although the number of treated patients is relatively small, responses have been observed in melanoma and renal cell carcinoma (RCC).

Here we summarize results from our phase I trial of TILs in patients with metastatic RCC and present data that characterize the cultured TILs in terms of their phenotype and cytolytic properties. Additional work defines the state of activation of TILs prior to culturing in recombinant IL-2 (rIL-2).

Materials and Methods

Clinical Studies with TILs

An ongoing clinical trial utilizing TILs with or without rIL-2 is underway, and patients with a minimal tumor burden (serum $Ca^{2+} < 11.0$ mg/dl, $\leq 30\%$ hepatic involvement on computerized tomography) and metastatic RCC are eligible. Therapy consists of either TILs alone or with escalating doses of rIL-2 (1.0, 3.0, 4.5×10^6 U/m^2). TILs were infused on days 1 and 8, and the rIL-2 was given for 2 weeks as a continuous infusion (days 1–5, 8–12). Cyclophosphamide was added at

[1] The Cleveland Clinic Foundation, One Clinic Center, 9500 Euclid Avenue, Cleveland, OH 44195, USA

F.M.J. Debruyne et al. (Eds.)
Immunotherapy of Renal Cell Carcinoma

dose level IVa to inhibit suppression that might be present, as had been suggested by others [11, 12].

Source of rIL-2

The rIL-2 (NSC 60064) was kindly provided by Hoffman-LaRoche, Inc. (Nutley, NJ), and supplied by the National Cancer Institute. It was produced in an *E. coli* expression vector from cloned human DNA using recombinant DNA technology. It had a specific activity between 5 and 15×10^6 U/mg protein and contained < 0.312 EU/10^6 NU of endotoxin.

Human Renal Cell Carcinoma TIL Isolation and Expansion In Vitro

The kidneys obtained from nephrectomies were perfused with 500 ml of Hanks balanced salt solution (Whittaker Bioproducts, Walkersville, MD) to remove extraneous blood. The primary and metastatic tumors were processed as previously described [14].

TILs were placed in gas-permeable bags containing either Aim V media (Gibco Laboratories) or ex Vivo 10 media (Whittaker Bioproducts) at a total cell concentration of 2.5×10^5/ml supplemented with 1000 U/ml of rIL-2 and incubated at 37°C in 5% CO_2 and 95% humidity. TIL cultures were fed on day 10 with fresh media and rIL-2 and then fed as needed to keep the cell concentration at 2.5×10^5/ml. TILs used for adoptive therapy were harvested using the SteriCell system (E.I. Dupont De Nemones & Co.).

Isolation of Tumor Targets

After a 4-h incubation period in collagenase and DNase, $1–2 \times 10^6$ tumor cells were placed in primaria grade tissue culture flasks (Becton Dickinson, Oxnard, CA) and cultured for a short term as previously described [14]. These short-term cultures represented RCC as was demonstrated by morphologic examination and immunostaining with antibodies to renal tissue associated antigens, Uro 2, as well as to cytoplasmic cytokeratin of epithelial cells AE1/3. When sufficient cells were available, growth in nude mice was demonstrated for the short-term cultured tumors.

Previously, we showed that rIL-2-expanded TILs from RCC were cytotoxic for uncultured autologous and allogeneic renal cell tumors [5]. Here we find that the same degree of lysis can be detected from TILs when short-term cultures of RCC are used as targets.

Daudi cells and the RCC line RC2 [15] were maintained in complete RPMI 1640 media (Whittaker Bioproducts) [14] and used as targets for cytotoxicity studies. All cell lines were periodically tested and found to be free of mycoplasma infection.

Isolation of $CD4^+$ and $CD8^+$ TILs

Anti-CD8 (IOT8) and anti-CD4 (IOT4) antibody coated beads (Amac, Inc., Westbrook, MA) were used to select positively for $CD8^+$ and $CD4^+$ cells, respectively. TILs cultured with rIL-2 were incubated at a 4:1 bead to cell ratio for 30 min at 4°C with gentle agitation every 5 min. The immediate negative cells (nonadherent) were separated using a BioMag Separator (Advanced Magnetics, Cambridge, MA). The cells with beads attached were washed twice with RPMI 1640 (Whittaker Bioproducts, Walkersville, MD), pipetted vigorously, and put in culture with Aim V media (Gibco, Grand Island, NY) and 1000 U/ml rIL-2. After 1–5 days, $CD8^+$ as well as $CD4^+$ cells were separated from the beads using BioMag Separator. The isolated $CD4^+$ and $CD8^+$ TILs were greater than 92% pure.

Cytolytic Activity

Detection of lytic activity was performed using 4- and 18-h ^{51}Cr release assay [14]. Various concentrations of cultured cells were added to U-bottom, 96-well plates to achieve effector to target cell ratios of 25:1 down to 0.78:1 (6 dilutions). In all the 4- and 18-h ^{51}Cr release assays the spontaneous release was never greater than 20%. Cytolytic activity was expressed as lytic units per 10^6 mononuclear cells tested as determined from linear regression analysis of dose-response curves in which the natural log of the number of effectors is plotted against percent specific lysis. One lytic unit was defined as the number of effector cells required to produce 15% specific lysis of 5×10^3 target cells in a 4 (and 18) h period.

Three Color Immunocytometry

Immunocytometric analysis of cultured TILs was performed as previously described [14]. Fluoroscein isothiocyanate (FITC), phycoerythrin, and biotin conjugated monoclonal antibodies were employed to identify phenotypically and quantitate lymphocytic subsets. Antibody titers were adjusted according to the fluorescence sensitivity of the flow cytometer (FACScan/BD) employed. Isotypic controls for each particular subclass of immunoglobulin and system employed were utilized to allow for the most accurate delineation of positive and autofluorescent populations and to control for nonspecific binding by a particular subclass of immunoglobulin.

Table 1. Patients at each dose level treated by tumor-infiltrating lymphocytes

Dose level	Number of patients treated/entered	rIL-2 (U/m^2) (D1–5 D8–12)	CTX (25 mg/kg) (D1)
I	3/4	0	0
II	5/6	1×10^6	0
III	5/9	3×10^6	0
IV	3/4	4.5×10^6	0
IVa	3/3	$4.5 \times 10^6 4$	4

rIL-2, recombinant interleukin-2; *CTX*, cyclophosphamide; *D*, day of administration

Results

Clinical Study

Some 26 patients with metastatic RCC (Table 1) were entered into the study with the following eligibility criteria: performance status (ECOG) 0–1; adequate hematologic, renal, and hepatic function; absence of significant cardiac disease or pulmonary disease (left ventricular ejection fraction $\geq$ 50%) (FEV > 2.01); and absence of CNS metastases. Prior chemotherapy, immunotherapy, or hormonal therapy led to disqualification. Radiotherapy within 4 weeks of entry into the study was allowed. Nineteen patients were subsequently treated.

Patients were monitored daily for toxicities which were graded according to the NCI Common Toxicity Criteria. These were modified to allow continued therapy with rIL-2 and grade 3 toxicity as follows:

1) pulmonary – dyspnea at rest requiring supplemental O_2 or ventilatory support;
2) cardiac – any occurrence of angina or ventricular arrhythmia;
3) vascular – hypotension unresponsive to phenylephrine hydrochloride;
4) CNS – any neurotoxicity; and
5) serum creatinine > 5 mg/dl and/or total bilirubin > 5 mg/dl.

All patients tolerated the TIL infusion without significant toxicities. Varying degrees of fever, chills, fatigue, anorexia, and nausea were experienced by all patients, but these were transient. Dose-limiting toxicity was seen at dose level IV (rIL-2 4.5×10^6 U/m^2), including refractory hypotension (2/6), respiratory distress (3/6), and mental status change (1/6). All toxicities resolved within 24–72 h after the discontinuation of the rIL-2 infusion, and no additional toxicity was attributable to the administration of cyclophosphamide. No objective clinical responses have been observed, although one patient with a soft tissue metastasis was noted to have a minor regression of the tumor.

Table 2. Tumor-infiltrating lymphocyte expansion

Sourse of tumor	*n*	Number of cells infused		Fold increase	
		Median	Range	Median	Range
Primary	13	3.18×10^{10}	$1.37 \times 10^{9} - 2.24 \times 10^{12}$	35.8	2.6–6229
Metastatic	6	1.47×10^{10}	$1.24 \times 10^{9} - 3.30 \times 10^{12}$	119.2	4.4–251 281

Primary and metastatic tumors were digested with an enzyme cocktail as described in materials and methods

Table 3. Phenotype of tumor-infiltrating lymphocyte (TIL) infused (percentage of lymphocytes at first infusion)

Phenotype	*n*	Percentage positive lymphocytes		
		Mean	Median	Range
$CD3^+$	18	77.8	86.5	27.8–99.6
$CD56^+$	18	39.2	32.0	6.8–87.2
$CD3^+CD25^+HLADR^+$	18	49.9	59.0	0.6–91.8
$CD8^+CD3^+CD4^-$	18	42.8	37.0	0.0–97.1
$CD8^-CD3^+CD4^+$	18	23.6	13.2	0.0–96.5

Cultured TILs were analyzed by three color immunocytometry

Growth of TILs in rIL-2

Growth characteristics of TILs are shown in Table 2. TILs from most primary and metastatic RCC could be expanded to sufficient numbers for infusion. There was inadequate growth in two cultures and contamination in three others. The level of TIL expansion in vitro was not associated with the tumor site (metastatic vs. primary) degree of initial infiltrate, or phenotype of TIL. Nineteen patients were treated with TIL ± rIL-2 according to the schedule shown in Table 1. The total number of TILs infused per patient ranged from 1.2×10^9 to 3.3×10^{12}, and in 8/18 patients $> 1 \times 10^{11}$ cells were infused.

Phenotypes of Cultured TILs

The phenotypes of the cultured TILs in 18 patients are presented in Table 3. In 14/18 patients > 70% were T cells with a $CD3^+$ phenotype. In the remaining 4 patients, the cells were predominantly $CD56^+$($Leu19^+$). In 2 patients, cells with the phenotype of natural killer (NK) cells ($CD3^-CD56^+CD8^-$ or $CD3^-CD16a^+CD56^+$) predominated. Therefore, initial analysis demonstrates that cultured TILs are predominantly T cells but are extremely heterogeneous in their phenotypes. NK cells

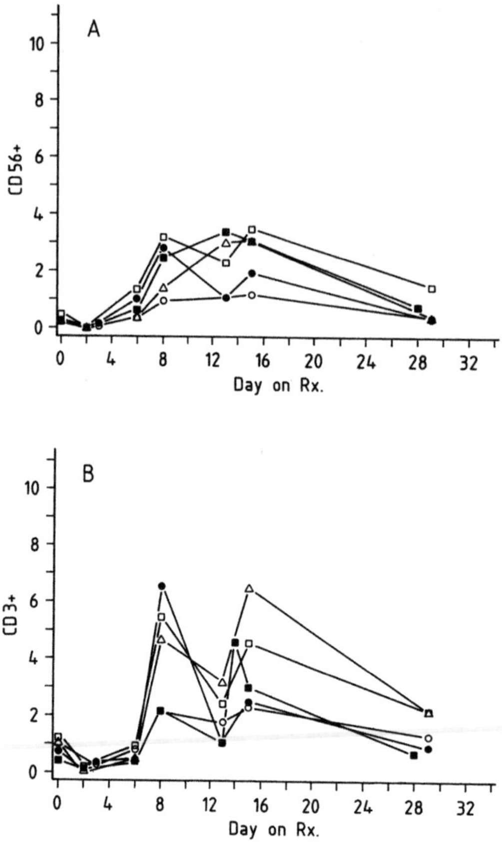

Fig. 1A,B. Three color flow analysis was conducted on peripheral blood lymphocytes before, during, and after dose level III therapy. **A** Changes in CD56$^+$; **B** changes in CD3$^+$

rarely predominate in culture although some preparations contain a significant number of these cells.

Changes in the Peripheral Blood of TIL + IL-2 Treated Patients

Lymphocyte subsets in the peripheral blood (PBL) of patients were analyzed by three color flow cytometry before, during, and after therapy. At dose level I no significant changes from baseline were observed; however, at other dose levels, significant increases in CD3$^+$ cells, CD56$^+$ cells, and activated CD3$^+$ (CD25$^+$HLADR$^+$) cells were observed. Figure 1 shows the data for patients at dose level III. These changes in CD3$^+$ and CD56$^+$ cells are different from those reported for rIL-2 alone or in rIL-2 and rHuIFNα2a studies (data not shown). At dose levels above

Table 4. Lytic activity of $CD4^+$ tumor-infiltrating lymphocytes (TILs) in 18-h ^{51}Cr release assay[a]

	Tumor targets LU/10^6 [b]		
Experiments	Autologous	Allogenic	Renal cell 2
1	0.6	ND	0.0
2	108.0	11.8	0.0
3	353.0	164.0	4.4
4	241.0	ND	5.8
5	0.0	1.1	0.0
6	3.6	ND	0.0

[a] Cytolytic $CD4^+$ TILs isolated using antibody-coated beads and tested in an 18-h ^{51}Cr release assay
[b] Based on 15% lysis derived from the following effector to target ratios – 25:1, 12.5:1, 6.25:1, 3.125:1, 1.562:1, 0.781:1
LU, lytic units; *ND*, not determined

I, increases in PBL lytic activity were observed against Daudi and the autologous tumor targets in patients treated with TILs and rIL-2 (data not shown).

Cytolytic Activity of Cultured TILs

The majority of TIL cultures used for infusion displayed non-MHC restricted lytic activity (5; data not shown). To define the effector cells present in TILs, the cytolytic activity of the two predominant TIL subsets, $CD3^+CD4^+$ and $CD3^+CD8^+$, was compared with that of the $CD56^+$ populations. In a 4-h ^{51}Cr release assay the $CD4^+$ and $CD8^+$ TILs that were isolated with the biomagnetic beads showed minimal lytic activity whereas unseparated cells exhibited significant levels of non-MHC-restricted cytotoxicity [14, 16]. Most of the lytic activity seen in the 4-h assay with unseparated TILs appeared to be related to the presence of $CD56^+$ populations [16]. Cell sorting experiments verified that the $CD56^+$ populations were responsible for most of the lytic activity at 4 h even though $CD3^+CD56^-$ cells represented the predominant cell type. $CD5^+CD56^-$ TILs displayed minimal lytic activity whereas the $CD5^-CD56^+$ and to a lesser degree the $CD5^+CD56^+$ cells were lytic for the autologous and allogeneic tumor targets [16].

Further analysis of the $CD4^+$ and $CD8^+$ TIL subsets revealed that both have antitumor activity for RCC. In an 18-h ^{51}Cr release assay four out of six $CD4^+$ TILs enriched by biomagnetic beads were lytic for the autologous tumor (Table 4). Even though the lytic activity was not specific, in some cases the greatest lysis mediated by $CD4^+$ TILs was observed against the autologus tumor. Of the three $CD8^+$ TIL subsets analyzed for lysis of the autologous tumor, two demonstrated lytic activity at 18 h but not at 4 h (data not shown).

Table 5. Enhancement of lysis by pretreatment of renal cell carcinoma tumor targets with interferon-γ and tumor necrosis factor-α[a]

		Cytolytic activity[b]	
Experiment	Cells	Untreated	Treated
1	Unseparated	0.5	60.9
	$CD8^+$	4.2	76.8
	$CD4^+$	0.6	9.4
2	Unseparated	0.8	55.0
	$CD8^+$	5.0	69.7
	$CD4^+$	7.0	6.7

[a] Tumor treated with 1000 U/ml IFN-γ and 1000 U/ml TNF-α for 72 h

[b] Cytolytic activity was determined in a 4-h ^{51}Cr release assay, and the results are presented in lytic units /10^6 cells

Additional studies showed that these $CD3^+CD56^-$ TILs can mediate lysis of autologous RCC in 4 h provided tumor targets are pretreated with a combination of tumor necrosis factor alpha (TNF-α) and IFNγ (Table 5) [11]. Our results are in agreement with those of Stotter et al. [17] who showed that pretreatment with IFNγ and TNF-α increased the susceptibility of tumor cells to lysis by TILs but not by lymphokine-activated killer (LAK) cells. Here we extend their observation and show that most of the lytic response against the cytokine-treated targets was mediated by $CD3^+CD8^+$ and to a much lesser degree by $CD3^+CD4^+$ TILs from RCC (Table 5). The lytic response observed with the treated targets was not restricted to the autologous tumor since TILs lysed allogeneic RCC that were pretreated with this cytokine combination (data not shown). Collectively, these results suggest that both $CD4^+$ and $CD8^+$ T cells from RCC TILs which lack CD56 have cytolytic activity.

State of TIL Activation In Situ

In an attempt to determine whether TILs represent a population of T cells that have been exposed to antigen and are part of the local host immune response to tumor, we examined their state of activation. CD29 (detected by mAb 4B4), a 135 kDa surface protein [18], and CD45RO (detected by mAb UCHL1), a 180 kDa component of the leukocyte common antigen (LCA) [19–21], have been shown to be expressed on activated lymphocytes but not on nonactivated resting lymphocytes. The expression of CD29 and CD45RO is increased on T cells following activation with phytohemagglutinin (PHA) or antigen [22]. Concomitant with the

Table 6. Tumor-infiltrating lymphoctes (TILs) are depleted of T cells expressing the naive marker (CD45RA) and enriched for those expressing the permanent activation marker (CD45RO)

	Percentage positive lymphocytes	
	$CD3^{+}CD45RO^{+}CD45RA^{-}$	$CD3^{+}CD45RO^{-}CD45RA^{+}$
TIL	42.4 ± 5.7	5.3 ± 1.8
PBL	30.9 ± 2.7	25.7 ± 1.8

Paired peripheral blood lymphocyte (PBL) and TIL samples from 17 patients with renal cell carcinoma were analyzed by three color immunocytometry on the day of study. Cells were labelled with antibodies to CD45RA (leu18), CD45RO (UCHL1), and CD3 (Leu4) and analyzed in a FACScan. The results are presented as the mean (+SE) of the percentage of positively stained lymphocytes

increase in the surface expression of these two markers is a decrease in the expression of CD45RA (formerly CD45R), the 220 kDa component of the LCA, a surface structure associated with naive cells [22]. Included was an analysis of TILs expressing transient activation markers such as the gp 55 protein of IL-2R (CD25) and HLA-DR. Using three color flow cytometry we showed that TILs are indeed composed of a high percentage of activated T cells. Most of TILs did not express CD25, whereas a significant number (28%) expressed HLA-DR (data not shown). An analysis of the permanent markers revealed that the ratio of activated versus nonactivated T cells within human RCC differs significantly from what is observed in the peripheral blood. Based on the expression of CD45RO in TILs, there were eight times more activated than nonactivted $CD3^{+}$ cells compared with peripheral blood where the number of activated and nonactivated cells were comparable (ratio $\simeq$ 1:1) (Table 6). Concomitant with the increase in activated cells was a significant decrease in naive cells (CD45RA) within the tumor.

Discussion

Phase I/II trials of TILs in RCC and melanoma have been completed, and Rosenberg et al. have reported a 50% response rate in patients with melanoma using a combination of TILs, rIL-2, and cyclophosphamide [11, 12]. This response rate appears higher than those observed with high-dose rIL-2 alone, suggesting that the TILs are mediating an effect in vivo. However, smaller numbers of patients with RCC treated with TILs have been reported. To date only four such patients have been included [12], and one patient has had a response. Kradin et al. [13] using a different schedule of TIL administration (three times per week $\times 7$ doses) and a constant dose infusion schedule of rIL-2 for 13 days reported 2/7 responses in patients with RCC and 3/13 responses in patients with melanoma.

In our study, 19 patients were treated, and one minor regression has been observed. It is difficult to compare our results with the previously reported studies since various schedules of rIL-2 injection, TIL administration, and cyclophosphamide application have been employed as well as different methods of TIL activation. Furthermore, the heterogeneity of the infused cells makes analysis of efficacy difficult. In our studies, detailed three color flow cytometry demonstrates the extreme heterogeneity of TILs between patients as well as between infusion on days 1 and 8. Thus, the admixture of cells may be a major contributing factor in abrogating or diluting the activity of any particular subset in the bulk population of TILs.

These studies also showed that TILs cultured in high doses of rIL-2 for infusion contain several populations with potential cytolytic activity. Most of the lytic activity as seen in a 4-h assay was due to LAK cells ($CD3^-CD56^+$, $CD3^+CD56^+$) [23], which is in agreement with what has been reported for TILs from head/neck and ovarian tumors [24, 25]. We show here that $CD3^+CD56^-$ cells, which represent a significant portion of the cultured TILs, do have antitumor activity that can be detected by using either an 18-h ^{51}Cr release assay or by pretreating tumor targets with cytokines. The functional heterogeneity of cultured TILs was also illustrated at the clonal level where it was found that a significant number of $CD8^+$ TIL clones were not lytic whereas other displayed cytotoxic activity at either 4 or 18 h (Finke et al., manuscript in preparation). Results presented here suggest that $CD8^+$ and to a lesser degree $CD4^+$ TILs which do not appear to be cytolytic can mediate lysis of cytokine-treated tumor target cells. Thus, some RCC may not be sensitive to the cytolytic activity of TILs, but such cells can be made susceptible by exposure to cytokines. Whether pretreatment with TNF-α/IFNγ would improve the therapeutic activity of RCC TILs is not known but is being addressed.

Evidence presented here suggests that TILs in RCC represent a local host response to tumor. This hypothesis was supported by the fact that most TILs have the phenotype of antigen-primed resting T cells. A significant percentage of the TILs express $CD45RO^+$ and lack the transient marker CD25 (IL-2R). Whether a portion of the activated cells display immunological memory for RCC is being tested. Studies are also in progress to develop procedures for isolating and expanding tumor-specific T cells from the activated population of TILs. It may be that the use of T-cell subsets with specific helper and lytic activity will represent an improvement in the use of TILs for adoptive immunotherapy in RCC and other tumors.

References

1. Vose BM, Moore M (1985) Human tumor-infiltrating lymphocytes: a marker of host response. Seminars in Hematology 11:17
2. Whiteside TL, Miescher S, Hurlimann J, Moretta L, Fliedner V von (1986) Separation, phenotyping and limiting dilution analysis of T-lymphocytes infiltrating human solid tumors. Int J Cancer 37:803
3. Itoh K, Tilden AB, Balch CM (1986) Interleukin-2 activation of cytotoxic T-lymphoctes infiltrating into human metastatic melanomas. Can Res 46:3011-3017
4. Muul LM, Spiess PJ, Director EP, Rosenberg SA (1987) Identification of specific cytolytic immune response against autologous tumor in humans bearing malignant melanoma. J Immunol 138:989
5. Finke JH, Tubbs R, Connely B, Pontes E, Montie J (1988) Tumor infiltrating lymphocytes in patients with renal cell carcinoma. In: Battisto J, Plate J, Shearer G (eds) Cytotoxic T cells; biology and relevance to disease. New York Academy of Science, pp 387–394
6. Belldegrun A, Muul LM, Rosenberg SA (1988) Interleukin-2 expanded tumor-infiltrating lymphocytes in human renal cell cancer: isolation, characterization, and antitumor activity. Cancer Res 48:206–214
7. Itoh K, Platsoucas CD, Balch CM (1988) Autologous tumor-specific cytotoxic T lymphocytes in the infiltrate of human metastatic melanomas. Activation by interleukin-2 and autologous tumor cells and involvement of the T cell receptor. J Exp Med 168:1419–1441
8. Vose BM (1982) Quantitation of proliferative and cytotoxic precursor cells directed against human tumors: limiting dilution analysis in peripheral blood and at the tumor site. Int J Cancer 30:135
9. Rosenberg SA, Spiess P, Lafreniere R (1986) A new approach to the adoptive immunotherapy of cancer with infiltrating lymphocytes. Science 233:1318
10. Spiess PJ, Yang JC, Rosenberg SA (1987) In vivo antitumor activity of tumor-infiltrating lymphocytes expanded in recombinant interleukin-2. JNCI 75:1067
11. Rosenberg SA, Packard BS, Aebersold PM et al. (1988) Use of tumor-infiltrating lymphocytes and interleukin-2 in the immunotherapy of patients with metastatic melanoma. N Engl J Med 319:1676–1680
12. Topalian SL, Solomon D, Avis FF, Chang AE et al. (1988) Immunotherapy of patients with advanced cancer using tumor-infiltrating lymphocytes and recombinant interleukin-2: a pilot study. J Clin Oncol 6:839–853
13. Kradin RL, Lazarus DS, Dubinett SM et al. (1984) Tumor-infiltrating lymphocytes and interleukin-2 in treatment of advanced cancer. Lancet 1:577–580
14. Alexander J, Rayman P, Edinger M et al. (1990) TIL from renal cell carcinoma: restimulation with tumor influences proliferation and cytolytic activity. Int J Cancer 45:119–124
15. Hashimura T, Tubbs R, Connelly R et al. (1989) Characterization of two cell lines with distinct phenotypes and genotypes established from a patient from renal cell carcinoma. Cancer Res 49:7064–7071
16. Finke JH, Rayman P, Alexander J et al. (1990) Characterization of the cytolytic activity of $CD4^+$ and $CD8^+$ TIL subsets in human renal cell carcinoma. Cancer Res 50:2363–2370
17. Stotter H, Wiebke EA, Tomita S et al. (1989) Cytokines alter target cell susceptibility to lysis. II Evaluation of tumor infiltrating lymphocytes. J Immunol 142:1767–1773
18. Morimoto C, Letvin NL, Boyd AW et al. (1985) The isolation and characterization of the human helper inducer T cell subset. J Immunol 134 (6):3762
19. Smith S, Brown MH, Rose D et al. (1986) Functional subsets of human helper-inducer cells defined by a new monoclonal antibody, UCHL1. Immunology 58:63

20. Workshop Antigen Designation (1989) J Immunol 143 (2):758
21. Terry LA, Brown MH, Beverley PCL (1988) The monoclonal antibody, UCHL1, recognizes a 180,000 MW component of the human leucocyte-common antigen CD45. Immunology 64:331
22. Sanders ME, Makgoba MW, Sharrow SO et al. (1988) Human memory T lymphoctes express increased levels of three cell adhesion molecules (LFA-3, CD2, and LFA-1) and three other molecules (UCHL1, CDw29, and PgP-1) and have enhanced IFN gamma production. J Immunol 140 (5):1401
23. Lanier LL, Le AM, Civin CI et al. (1986) The relationship of CD16 (Leu11) and Leu19 (NKH-1) antigen expression on human peripheral blood NK cells and cytotoxic T lymphocytes. J Immunol 136:4480–4486
24. Whiteside TL, Heo DS, Takagi S et al. (1988) Cytolytic antitumor effector cells in long-term cultures of human tumor-infiltrating lymphocytes in recombinant interleukin 2. Cancer Immunol Immunother 26:1
25. Heo DS, Whiteside TL, Kunbour A, Herberman RB (1988) Lymphocytes infiltrating human ovarian tumors I. Role of Leu-19 (NHH1)-positive recombinant IL 2-activted cultures of lymphocytes infiltrating human ovarian tumors.

Active Specific Immunotherapy in Renal Cell Carcinoma: Optimization

C.S. McCune[1]

Introduction

The requirements for effective cancer vaccines have gradually been worked out in experimental models over the past 15 years [1–3]. Many clinical trials in this field were initiated before this information was available or did not adhere to the methodologic requirements that had been found in the animal studies. As a consequence, there are several negative clinical investigations of active specific immunotherapy in which failure was a virtual certainty [4–6] when looked at in retrospect with regard to the requirements that have been identified in animal models. Some of the key requirements are as follows:

a) The tumor cells should be preserved in a viable form in those vaccines in which whole tumor cells are used, or each procedure toward a subcellular product must be carefully evaluated as the immunogenicity can be easily destroyed.
b) The cryopreservation procedure for storing tumor tissue or tumor cells for later use in a vaccine must be carefully evaluated and shown not to destroy the immunogenicity of the vaccine.
c) The use of an adjuvant is essential, but the adjuvant must be given at a predetermined optimal concentration. Tumor vaccines are considered to be weakly antigenic, and the use of an effective adjuvant is critical to success, but selection of the wrong dose can negate the adjuvant's role.
d) The dose of tumor cells or quantity of antigenic material is a critical factor, and when an inadequate dose is given, the immunologic effect will be lost.
e) The animal studies had predicted that the use of the patient's own tumor cells (autologous) would have the highest likelihood of success compared with allogeneic cells.

Indeed the initial successes in clinical studies have occurred with autologous cells. However, in the longer outlook, the use of allogeneic cell lines would have great practical advantages in the methods of production and standardization and in the ability to provide antigenic diversity in the vaccine.

[1] University of Rochester Medical Center, Medical Oncology Division,
601 Elmwood Avenue, Box 704, Rochester, NY 14642, USA

F.M.J. Debruyne et al. (Eds.)
Immunotherapy of Renal Cell Carcinoma

Table 1. Forms of cell mediated immunotherapy

	Vaccines for ASI	TILs with IL-2	LAK cells with IL-2	IL-2
Immune cells produced where?	In host	Ex vivo	Ex vivo	In host
Generates antigen-specific immune cells	Yes	Yes	No	No
Achieves immunologic memory	Yes	Possibly	No	No
Potential for responding to antigenic diversity	Autologous: difficult Allogeneic: very possible	Possible but difficult	Not antigen-specific	Not antigen-specific

ASI, active specific immunotherapy; *TILs*, tumor-infiltrating lymphocytes; *LAK*, lymphokine-activated killer; *IL-2*, interleukin-2.

Table 2. Practical considerations in comparison of treatments

	Vaccines for ASI	TILs with IL-2	LAK cells with IL-2	IL-2
Laboratory support required	Small	Large	Large	None
Hospitalization requirement	None	Yes	Yes	Yes and no
Requires patient tumor tissue	Autologous: Yes Allogeneic: No	Yes	No	No
Side effects	Minimal	Major	Major	Major

ASI, active specific immunotherapy; *TILs*, tumor-infiltrating lymphocytes; *LAK*, lymphokine-activated killer; *IL-2*, interleukin-2

The clinical trials of vaccines for active specific immunotherapy have had some success with three types of malignancy: renal carcinoma [7–12], colon carcinoma [13, 14], and malignant melanoma [15, 16].

Comparison of Active Specific Immunotherapy with Other Forms of Cell-Mediated Immunotherapy

The very interesting clinical investigations in recent years with lymphokine-activated killer (LAK) cells and tumor-infiltrating lymphocytes (TILs) have given a broader acceptance to the idea that immune cells can produce remissions of cancer. Although major shortcomings and problems remain, the reality that metastases have responded is established. This leads to the issue of which forms of cell-mediated immunotherapy have the greatest potential for further development. Tables 1 and

Table 3. Variable responses of metastases occurring in the same patient

	Complete response	Partial response	Stable	Progression	Total measurable metastases
Patient 1	18		4		22
Patient 5	4	1	1	3	9
Patient 6		1	1	2	4
Patient 13	2	1			3

2 compare four types of immunologic treatment; all have substantial evidence that they are cell-mediated, and all have produced remissions.

Two important considerations which recommend the vaccine approach are that the immune cells are generated in the host rather than ex vivo and that the immunologic response to vaccines leads to an immunologic memory. A long-lived, constantly circulating population of sensitized lymphocytes not dependent on IL-2 resulting from a vaccine is conceptually a much more desirable goal than the transient circulation of laboratory-produced effector cells requiring hospitalization levels of IL-2 or other cytokines for support.

Major Problems

Two central problems which must be dealt with so that the field of active specific immunotherapy can move forward are the following:

1. Selection of an antigen source which can both generate tumor rejecting immunity and deal with the antigenic diversity of the tumor.
2. The immune response to vaccines must be augmented to a level which is more consistently effective.

The problem of antigen diversity appears to be of great importance. Mixed responses in which some metastases regress while others do not are seen with each form of cell-mediated immunotherapy. Our experience with four patients suffering from metastatic renal carcinoma [8] is illustrated in Table 3.

Antigen Source

Options under consideration for cancer vaccines are shown in Table 4. The clinical studies which have succeeded in producing regressions of metastases or survival benefits in randomized trials have often employed autologous whole tumor cells [8, 9, 11–15], but an autologous vaccine of aggregated antigens also succeeded in the treatment of renal carcinoma [7]. Recently, an allogeneic lysate has succeeded as a vaccine for melanoma [16].

Table 4. Vaccine options for active specific immunotherapy

Autologous
Whole tumor cells
Aggregated antigens
Allogeneic
Whole tumor cells
Lysates
Virus-infected lysates
Supernatant tumor antigens
Extracted tumor antigens
Transfected tumor antigen genes expressed in vaccinia
Antigens represented by antiidiotype antibodies

A central issue which remains to be resolved in the development of cancer vaccines is whether autologous sources of antigens must be used or whether allogeneic sources can be substituted. This issue is illustrated by the two classic preclinical experiments illustrated in Tables 5 and 6, which have been repeated in many laboratories. The experiment by Law [18] suggested that each tumor has unique antigens or epitopes which produce highly specific cell-mediated immunity. The experiments by Economou [19] indicated that cross reactivity exists between murine tumors induced by the same carcinogen. The human studies thus far do not provide enough experience or data to determine whether an autologous or allogeneic source is preferable. The studies in renal carcinoma which have used autologous or allogeneic antigen sources are given in Table 7.

Augmenting the Response

We have been studying in an animal model the possibility that cytokines might be used to augment the immune response to vaccines [17]. An experiment with interleukin-1 which illustrates the potential contribution of these agents is shown in Table 8. Mice were immunized with a vaccine of radiated tumor cells on day 1 and received IL-1β or a peptide fragment of IL-1β by injection on days 1–8. On day 15 the mice were challenged with tumor. Both the peptide and the whole molecule of IL-1β were capable of significantly improving the effects of the vaccine.

In summary, two promising directions in which vaccines can potentially be significantly improved are (1) selection of an antigen source to deal with antigenic diversity and (2) the use of cytokines to augment the effectiveness of vaccines.

Table 5. Results of experiment suggesting uniqueness of tumor antigens [18]

Immunized with	Challenged with[a]				
	1	3	4	5	7
Tumor 1	18/18	NCR	NCR	NCR	NCR
Tumor 3	NCR	17/18	NCR	ND	NCR
Tumor 4	NCR	NCR	16/16	NCR	NCR
Tumor 5	NCR	NCR	NCR	9/25	ND
Tumor 7	NCR	NCR	NCR	ND	25/27

[a] Results are tumor-free/total
NCR, no cross reactivity

Table 6. Results of experiment indicating cross reactivity between murine tumors induced by the same carcinogen [19]

Immunized with	Challenged with[a]				
	2	3	6	7	10
Tumor 2	9/10	1/8	[8/8]	0/8	[7/8]
Tumor 3	1/9	9/9	[8/8]	2/10	[8/8]
Tumor 6	0/10	0/10	8/8	2/10	0/8
Tumor 7	1/10	1/8	[8/8]	8/8	1/8
Tumor 10	[6/10]	[5/10]	[8/8]	1/11	9/9

[a] Results are tumor-free/total

Table 7. Vaccine trials for renal carcinoma

Author	McCune [8, 9]	Tykka [7]	Neidhart [10]	Adler [11]	Scharfe [12]
Antigen source	Autologous	Autologous	Allogeneic	Autologous	Autologous
Vaccine type	Whole cells	Aggregated antigens	Aggregated antigens	Whole cells	Whole cells
Disease stage	Metastatic	Metastatic	Metastatic	Adjuvant and metastatic	Metastatic
Results	Partial remissions	Partial remissions	Partial remissions	Trend in survival advantage	Complete and partial remissions

Table 8. Adjuvant effect of interleukin (IL)-1β or the peptide fragment 163-171

Group	Vaccine	Peptide of IL-1β(ng)	IL-1β(ng)	Mean survival (days ± SE)[a]	Tumor-free/ total	(%)[a]	Percentage weight change
1	–	–	–	14.90 ± 1.02	0/10	(0)	+6
2	3×10^5 TC	–	–	17.00 ± 0.97	0/10	(0)	+5
3	3×10^5 TC	360 × 8d	–	17.00 ± 0.68	0/10	(0)	+5
4	3×10^5 TC	3600 × 8d	–	24.90 ± 3.50*	3/10	(30)	+4
5	3×10^5 TC	36000 × 8d	–	22.60 ± 3.01	2/10	(20)	+3
6	3×10^5 TC	100000 × 8d	–	29.80 ± 3.69**	5/10	(50)**	+1
7	3×10^5 TC	–	120 × 8d	33.80 ± 3.66***	7/10	(70)****	+6
8	3×10^5 TC	–	360 × 8d	40.00 ± 0.00***	10/10	(100)*****	+0.6

[a] Statistical comparisons with group 2 are indicated

* $P < 0.05$, ** $P < 0.01$, *** $P < 0.001$, **** $P = 0.001$, ***** $P < 0.0004$

TC, tumor cells; *d*, days

References

1. Bartlett GL, Zbar B (1972) Tumor-specific vaccine containing mycobacterium bovis and tumor cells: safety and efficacy. J Natl Cancer Inst 48:1709–1726
2. Scott MT (1975) Potentiation of the tumor-specific immune response by Corynebacterium parvum. J Natl Can Inst 55:65–72
3. Hanna MG, Peters LC (1981) Morphological and functional aspects of active specific immunotherapy of established pulmonary metastases in guinea pigs. Cancer Res 41:4001–4009
4. Hudson CN, McHardy JE, Curling OM et al. (1976) Active specific immunotherapy for ovarian cancer. Lancet 7991:877–879
5. Newlands ES, Oon CJ, Roberts JT et al. (1976) Clinical trial of combination chemotherapy and specific active immunotherapy in disseminated melanoma. Br J Cancer 34:174–179
6. Gray BN, Walker C, Andrewartha L et al. (1988) Melbourne trial of adjuvant immunotherapy in operable large bowel cancer. Aust NZ J Surg 58:43–46
7. Tykka H, Oravisto KJ, Lehtonen T et al. (1978) Active specific immunotherapy of advanced renal-cell carcinoma. Eur Urol 4:250–258
8. McCune CS, Schapira DV, Henshaw EC (1981) Specific immunotherapy of advanced renal carcinoma: evidence for the polyclonality of metastases. Cancer 47:1984–1987
9. Sahasrabudhe DM, deKernion JB, Pontes JE et al. (1986) Specific immunotherapy with suppressor function inhibition for metastatic renal cell carcinoma. J Biol Resp Mod 5:581–594
10. Neidhart JA, Gagen M, Young D, Wise H (1983) A randomized study of polymerized tumor antigen admixed with adjuvant for therapy of renal cancer. Proc Am Soc Clin Oncol 2:49
11. Adler A, Gillon G, Lurie H et al. (1987) Active specific immunotherapy of renal cell carcinoma patients: a prospective randomized study of hormono-immuno-versus hormonotherapy. Preliminary report of immunological and clinical aspects. J Biol Resp Mod 6:610–624
12. Scharfe T, Muller S, Riedmiller H et al. (1989) Immunotherapy of metastasizing renal cell carcinoma. Urol Int 44:1–4
13. Hoover HC, Surdyke M, Dangel RB et al. (1984) Delayed cutaneous hypersensitivity to autologous tumor cells in colorectal cancer patients immunized with an autologous tumor cell: Bacillus Calmette-Guerin vaccine. Cancer Res 44:1671–1676
14. Hoover HC, Surdyke MG, Dangel RB et al. (1985) Prospectively randomized trial of adjuvant active-specific immunotherapy for human colorectal cancer. Cancer 55:1236–1243
15. Berd D, Maguire HC, Mastrangelo MJ (1986) Induction of cell-mediated immunity to autologous melanoma cells and regression of metastases after treatment with a melanoma cell vaccine preceded by cyclophosphamide. Cancer Res 46:2572–2577
16. Mitchell MS, Kan-Mitchell J, Kempf RA et al. (1988) Active specific immunotherapy for melanoma: phase I trial of allogeneic lysates and a novel adjuvant. Cancer Res 48:5883–5893
17. McCune CS, Marquis DM (1990) Interleukin-1 as an adjuvant for active specific immunotherapy in a murine tumor model. Cancer Res 50:1212–1215
18. Law LS (1980) Changes in tumor-specific antigen expression during passage in vitro and in vivo of newly derived methylcholanthrene-induced sarcomas of Balb/C mice. Int J Cancer 25:251–259
19. Economou GC, Takeichi N, Boone CW (1977) Common tumor rejection antigens in methylcholanthrene-induced squamous cell carcinomas of mice detected by tumor protection and a radioisotopic footpad assay. Cancer Res 37:37–41

Subject Index

GPSR Compliance

The European Union's (EU) General Product Safety Regulation (GPSR) is a set of rules that requires consumer products to be safe and our obligations to ensure this.

If you have any concerns about our products, you can contact us on ProductSafety@springernature.com

In case Publisher is established outside the EU, the EU authorized representative is:

Springer Nature Customer Service Center GmbH
Europaplatz 3
69115 Heidelberg, Germany

Batch number: 10704713

Printed by Printforce, the Netherlands